Calmer, Easier, Hap

D0198719

ABOUT THE AUTHOR

Noël Janis-Norton graduated from teacher-training college at New York University. Her career as a learning and behaviour specialist spans more than forty years. She has been a classroom teacher, a special needs teacher and advisor, a tutor specialising in learning strategies, a head teacher and a parenting educator.

Noël is the founder and director of the Calmer, Easier, Happier Parenting Centre in London, which provides courses and consultations for parents of toddlers through teens.

A regular speaker at professional conferences, Noël has also been featured on numerous television and radio programmes. In addition to lecturing widely in the UK and the US, she also trains teachers and parenting practitioners in her unique and highly effective methods. She is the spokesperson for National Family Week and the parenting expert for Macaroni Kid (a popular website for parents in the US).

Through her seminars, courses and talks for parents, and through her books, CDs and DVDs, she has helped transform the lives of tens of thousands of families. Noël's most comprehensive book, *Calmer, Easier, Happier, Parenting*, was published in 2012.

Noël has two grown children, a foster daughter and six grandchildren.

Calmer, Easier, Happier Homework

Noël Janis-Norton

HODDER &
STOUGHTON

First published in Great Britain in 2013 by Hodder & Stoughton
An Hachette UK company

1

Copyright © Noël Janis-Norton 2013

The right of Noël Janis-Norton to be identified as the Author
of the Work has been asserted by her in accordance with
the Copyright, Designs and Patents Act 1988.

A CIP catalogue record for this title is available from the British Library

Trade Paperback ISBN 978 1 444 73027 2
Ebook ISBN 978 1 444 73029 6

Typeset by Hewer Text UK Ltd, Edinburgh
Printed and bound by Clays Ltd, St Ives plc

Hodder & Stoughton policy is to use papers that are natural, renewable
and recyclable products and made from wood grown in sustainable
forests. The logging and manufacturing processes are expected to
conform to the environmental regulations of the country of origin.

Hodder & Stoughton Ltd
338 Euston Road
London NW1 3BH

www.hodder.co.uk

This book is dedicated to all parents who are searching for ways to guide their children to fulfil their academic potential and to feel more successful.

CONTENTS

ACKNOWLEDGEMENTS

Many wise individuals and innovative organisations have influenced and enriched my work with families and schools. In addition to all my colleagues at 'Calmer, Easier, Happier Parenting', past and present, I would like to acknowledge:

Alfred Adler

Applied Behavioural Analysis

Dorothy Baruch

Tony Buzan

Julia Cameron

Dale Carnegie

Deepak Chopra

Dalai Lama

Edward de Bono

Rudolph Dreikurs

Carol Dweck

Adele Faber and Elaine Mazlish

Selma Fraiberg

Howard Gardiner

Haim Ginott

Torey Hayden

John Holt

Jill Janis

Susan Jeffers

Landmark Education

Lindamood-Bell Learning Process

Philip McGraw

Maria Montessori

Psychology of Vision

Jane Ross and Lee Janis

Barbara Sher

Sally Smith

Son-rise Programme

Benjamin Spock

Twelve-Step Programmes

Marianne Williamson

Michelle Garcia Winner

Rosalind Wiseman

My profound gratitude to my dear friends — you know who you are — for your love, encouragement and belief in me.

Special thanks to all the Calmer, Easier, Happier parents, whose honesty, enthusiasm for new ideas and determination to create Calmer, Easier, Happier families continues to inspire me and give me hope for the future.

My deepest appreciation to my children, Jessica, Jordan and Chloe for their unstinting love and support, and to my grandchildren Shaun, Anna, Cameron, Alexander, Zoey and Sophia for reminding me, again and again, of the potential of the human spirit.

FOREWORD

When Noël Janis-Norton asked if I'd write this Foreword, I wasn't sure it was a good idea. 'I hate homework,' I said decisively.

But then, as a confirmed fan of *Calmer, Easier, Happier Parenting*, I was interested in what she had to say. Could she convince a confirmed homework-hater like me that there is a calmer, easier, happier way to cope with the wretched stuff? As I waited for the manuscript to arrive, I ran over the reasons for my prejudice and found three main bones of contention.

First, as a primary teacher thirty-odd years ago, I'd discovered that dreaming up suitable homework tasks, then marking the efforts of thirty-odd children, took a lot of time and effort. What's more, some pupils habitually handed in scrappy, careless work, far below their natural potential, whilst others turned in faultless scripts that were obviously the product of far more sophisticated brains than their own. It seemed to me that, in both cases, homework was a waste not only of their time, but also of mine.

Then, when I left teaching and had a child of my own, there were further reasons for resentment. To a busy working mum, struggling to put a cooked meal on the table every evening, homework was just one more responsibility to cram into the day — an externally imposed reason to nag my daughter and another infringement on our family's rapidly decreasing leisure time.

Finally, as an author on child development in the modern world, I've become increasingly worried by the way adult concerns now press down on to children at an ever-younger age. Homework is clearly necessary once youngsters reach secondary school, but too much emphasis before they reach double figures can be counter productive. It cuts into the time available for other developmentally essential activities, such as playing (*real* play, not staring at screens), learning essential life skills with their family and socialising with their friends.

So it's been interesting to read Noël's book, with these memories and concerns rattling round my brain, and then to find myself nodding sagely at the recommendations and strategies it contains. With her usual clear-sightedness, she's identified the habit of 'getting on with the job' as one of *the* most essential life skills parents can help their children develop. Every child needs to learn — as calmly and easily as possible — that some things just have to be done, and the sooner one gets them done, the happier life is.

It's all too easy for parents, beset by myriad demands on their own time, to forget that such habits of mind require careful nurture. Presumably that's why some of my pupils all those years ago took no pride in their homework, while others sat back and let Mum or Dad do it for them. I suspect that, once these children reached secondary age, they lacked the time management skills and mental self-discipline required to take full advantage of educational opportunities.

On the other hand, the kids in my class who *did* learn to complete their homework independently (and, looking back, I must admit they were in the majority) were developing habits of mind and behaviour that would stand them in good stead throughout their school careers and, indeed, the whole of their lives. And, come to think of it, my own daughter didn't really need all that much nagging — as Noël brilliantly puts it, she eventually learned to treat homework as an unavoidable fact of life (like the weather) and just got on with it, leaving plenty of time to play with her friends and share in the life of our family. Presumably my husband and I can claim some credit for her development of self-regulatory powers, but back in the days before 'parenting' was invented, the strategies we used were very hit and miss. If we'd had Noël's book, I'm sure it would have been much, much easier.

However, in spite of all my sage nodding and agreement, after ten years of research into modern childhood I'm still convinced that very young children don't need formal 'homework'. In the first six years of life — while they're still developing the emotional, social, physical and cognitive foundations that underpin formal academic operations — they learn best through play. Plenty of active outdoor play helps them develop bodily coordination and control; creative indoor play nurtures imagination and problem-solving skills; stories, songs and rhymes develop their ear for language, and counting games and songs prepare their minds for maths. Play, as child development experts repeatedly tell us, is 'children's work' and parents who take a relaxed, playful attitude in these early years help their offspring lay sound foundations for 'getting on with the job' in the future.

Tragically, over the last thirty or so years as life has moved on at an increasingly crazy pace, it's become ever more difficult for parents — and children — to be truly relaxed and playful at home. A family surrounded by a constant barrage of screen-based entertainment and communication tends to become fragmented, with parents and children increasingly out of touch with each other. So their home is no longer run according to their own shared family values, but those of the media and market forces that generate this 'screen saturation'.

That's why I so admire the advice in *Calmer, Easier, Happier Parenting*. It shows modern parents how to take a warm but firm *authoritative* approach to child rearing, thus releasing families to enjoy their time together rather than wasting it in nagging, resentment and individualised, isolated screen-gazing. It allows children to feel secure in the rules and routines of a comfortable family life, valued for their own contribution in terms of agreed duties and chores, and loved by parents who clearly enjoy their company.

And it's why now, having read *Calmer, Easier, Happier Homework*, I also greatly admire Noël's advice on applying these techniques to transform homework into a manageable fact of life, and a way of developing children's self-discipline, self-reliance and self-esteem.

In fact, if I'd had a copy of this book thirty years ago, I probably wouldn't have spent so much time hating homework myself. I would have seen the point and learned how to manage it.

Sue Palmer, November 2012

PARTNERS IN EDUCATION: PARENTS, PUPILS AND TEACHERS

CHAPTER 1

WHAT'S HOMEWORK LIKE AT YOUR HOUSE?

Since you're interested in this book, I'm guessing that homework in your house doesn't feel good — for you or for your child. Here are some of the common complaints I hear from parents about homework:

I have to sit next to her the whole time or she just stares out of the window.

He says it's too hard before he's barely looked at it.

Trying to cope with three children's homework is driving me mad. They all need me at the same time.

He keeps telling me there's no homework, but that can't be true.

Homework issues lead to conflict in many families: parents nagging, children and teens ignoring or answering back disrespectfully, parents complaining and blaming and then children complaining and blaming.

Homework doesn't have to be hell. Homework doesn't even have to be a hassle. Homework does not need to be experienced, either by your child or by you, as a burden or as a restriction. It doesn't have to be a blight on your evenings and weekends, and it doesn't have to swallow up hours and hours of your children's time or your time. You and your child can enjoy homework!

However, this delightful state of affairs is not likely to ever come to pass if we leave it up to our children to manage their time, to organise their work or to motivate themselves to do their best. Homework that is enjoyable and productive is more likely to happen if parents commit to getting back in charge of the homework process rather than leaving it in the hands of children, who are by definition immature.

The thought of getting back in charge may seem very daunting, even impossible, especially if you are currently dealing with a lot of resistance, refusal or disrespect. But in fact, getting back in charge can be an enjoyable, exhilarating and relaxing experience. Being in charge and seeing things at home go the way you want them to (most of the time) is a lot more fun than feeling frustrated, possibly even despairing, when family life is not going according to your values.

When homework becomes enjoyable and productive (yes, it is possible!) everyone in the family can relax. Children have more guilt-free downtime. Parents have the satisfaction of seeing their children developing important habits that will stand them in good stead for the rest of their lives.

Problems with homework rarely occur in isolation. For example, many children put off starting their homework until too close to bedtime because they are glued to a screen for the earlier part of the evening. A tired child or teenager is not likely to do his best on his homework. His mind is sluggish, so thinking takes longer. He may end up staying up way past his bedtime to get his homework finished. Then in the morning, not surprisingly, he is reluctant to get out of bed. And when he does finally emerge, he may be grumpy and distractible.

Homework habits are fundamentally linked to these daily flashpoints: bedtimes, screen time, getting up in the mornings, after-school activities and socialising with friends. So if we want to improve our children's homework habits, it is not enough to think only about what is happening during the homework time. We need to treat our family as a little ecosystem and fine-tune how it functions throughout the day, rather than just focusing on the symptoms of homework hassles.

In this book I will be asking you to do certain things differently, to discipline yourself to do more and more of what works to establish enjoyable and productive homework habits and to do less and less of what gets us the opposite. I will however be focusing here solely on homework. In the companion volume, *Calmer, Easier, Happier Parenting*, I have gathered together a comprehensive toolkit of strategies that help parents guide children to become more and more cooperative, confident, motivated, self-reliant and considerate. In this book I will summarise these strategies and show how they can be applied specifically to homework.

One of the hallmarks of a system is that it produces a predictable result each time. This Calmer, Easier, Happier Homework system produces enjoyable and productive homework habits, as well as more confident children and more relaxed parents. This book will teach you how to work with your child confidently, how to stay calm and in charge, even when you are not yet feeling very confident. It will also show you how to break down into bite-sized chunks the tasks and skills that your child needs to master in order to do his best on his homework. This is important because we want children to be learning what they should be learning, rather than simply going through the motions while half of their brain is thinking about something else. This book can even teach you how to have fun doing all this.

The longest journey begins with a single step . . . again . . . and again.

CHAPTER 2

WHAT IS 'SCHOOL SUCCESS', AND WHY DOES IT MATTER SO MUCH?

As parents we want our children to fulfil their potential. We want to help our children to achieve everything that they are capable of achieving. And for most children a large part of the achievement that parents hope for is what we often call 'doing well at school'.

Parents know that 'school success' matters because:

- Children are naturally happier and more enthusiastic about life when their innate abilities are being fully used and stretched.
- Competence leads to confidence.
- The skills and habits learned at school will be very useful in later life, in the areas of further or higher education, work, relationships and leisure activities.
- School is a child's 'job', and society takes this job very seriously. Parents, relatives and even strangers ask:

How's school?

What are you studying?

How's your reading (or maths) coming along?

- Rightly or wrongly, a child is often judged, and soon comes to judge himself, according to his academic performance. Peers also notice and talk about school success and lack of success.

- When a child is not enjoying his 'job' or when he is consistently not doing well, he does not have the option, as we do, of switching jobs. He may suffer in silence, or he may suffer noisily, making problems for himself and for everyone around him.

If we allow our children to dawdle through their job half-heartedly, or to rush through it with poor attention to detail, they will not get much satisfaction from it. They will not be proud of themselves and will not learn all that they are capable of learning. When we require children to do their best, they feel more successful. They grow in confidence, motivation, self-reliance and consideration, as well as becoming more cooperative and less resistant. So for our sakes, as well as for our children's sakes, we need to help them 'learn how to learn'.

How can we help our children to be successful at school? How can we help them to enjoy challenges and to take pride in doing their best? To achieve these aims we need to consistently guide our children into useful habits. This is where homework comes in:

- Productive homework habits enable children to get the most out of their homework.
- Your child will take his homework habits with him into school.
- Homework is something parents can influence greatly.

Children generally act as if the purpose of homework is simply to get it over with! As adults, we know that homework can serve one or more of the following very important purposes:

- Practising, revising or memorising in order to reinforce what has been learned
- Exploring a new aspect of a topic
- Establishing productive work habits

In addition, homework can keep parents aware of:

- The subject matter being taught
- The school's standards
- How well the child is mastering the subject matter and achieving the school's standards

Many parents worry because they do not know how to bring out the best in their children. We have all seen how even a very bright child can drift into becoming an underachiever if he is not guided to develop good habits and sound basic skills. One distraught, confused father commented, 'I don't have a clue how to help my son get back on track. It feels like my wife and I are sitting helplessly on the sidelines as our boy digs himself deeper and deeper into bad habits.'

Thankfully, a child who finds learning or concentrating more difficult than most can be successful, and feel successful, if he receives the teaching and training that is right for his kind of brain. A child or teenager who has been taught efficient school success skills knows how to learn and therefore enjoys learning more. He has the tools to fulfil his brain's potential. If his potential is very high, we can expect him to master knowledge and skills at a high level. If his potential is more limited, he will find the learning process harder, slower or more frustrating. He may never be an academic high-flyer, but he can still fulfil his own potential.

The skills needed for school success

The basic academic skills

- Listening
- Speaking
- Reading
- Writing
- Numeracy

Positive attitudes (these are also skills, and they can be learned and honed)

- Enthusiasm
- Motivation
- Cooperation
- Curiosity
- Confidence
- Self-reliance
- Impulse-control
- Doing one's best
- Patience
- Perseverance
- Consideration

Useful habits

- Following instructions immediately
- Accepting correction and being willing to learn from it
- Practising new skills until they come easily and automatically

- Not expecting teachers to overlook minor problems and mistakes; not expecting teachers to bend the rules
- Using your common sense and thinking about solutions, rather than about problems
- Paying attention to details
- Assuming there is something to be learned from every situation
- Making a good impression by acting friendly, interested, polite, respectful and considerate, even when you don't feel like it
- Accepting praise, and giving yourself credit for improving

All these skills and habits can be learned. And it is the job of parents, not of teachers, to make sure that our children learn these skills and then practise them until they are habitual. Homework is the tool that parents can use to help children and teens learn these skills and habits and achieve their potential.

CHAPTER 3

WHY SCHOOLS BY THEMSELVES CANNOT HELP ALL PUPILS TO FULFIL THEIR POTENTIAL

There are several important reasons why parents cannot just sit back and expect teachers to do the job of training children in the all-important skills that lead to school success.

A great deal of research has been done about learning styles (strengths and weaknesses). Researchers know much more than they did even ten years ago about the relative effectiveness of different teaching styles. We now know, in theory, how to help every child to achieve his potential! But it can take a long time for research findings to become a reality in the classroom.

Teachers are exposed to new teaching methods mostly through in-service training. This is often delivered by lecturers who have not had recent experience of the harsh realities of the classroom. Without intending to, these lecturers may paint an unrealistically rosy picture of the school system, implying that new strategies will be easy to put into practice. The initial response of teachers to hearing about new strategies may be enthusiasm and excitement. But this can quickly sour because they are often expected to implement new ideas based only on a one-day course, and without effective, consistent support from their senior leadership team. Because of this, many useful strategies fall by the wayside, and teachers often end up feeling disillusioned.

Even when teachers do understand what a particular child needs in order to fulfil his potential, schools may not be able to provide what is needed, due to a shortage of funding. For example, in almost every classroom there will be a few children who need a very different kind of learning environment. They need individualised, skilled instruction and very quiet, purposeful, calm surroundings. These pupils may be too distractible, too self-conscious or too easily upset to stay focused on their work in a busy, noisy classroom.

Even pupils with an acknowledged, assessed learning disability and an official statement of special educational needs are likely to be receiving only a small fraction of what they would need in order to <u>really</u> achieve what they are capable of achieving.

Any pupil who is experiencing difficulties will learn more successfully and will feel more confident (and as a consequence will also behave more maturely) when he is given plenty of <u>time</u> to master a topic or skill before being expected to move on to the next level of difficulty. A great deal of schoolwork is sequential. Each new skill or topic is most easily learned and remembered when it is sitting on a solid foundation of previously mastered skills and information. When a pupil has not mastered certain basic skills and facts, any subsequent learning will be like building on sand. The structure is bound to be shaky.

But in the classroom more <u>time</u> is often not available to the child who needs it. It is easy to understand why teachers move the whole class on as soon as the majority of the pupils have shown that they are ready. The needs of the majority who are coping and learning seem to outweigh the needs of the few who are struggling. But the inescapable fact is that in every class there will be some children who need lessons that progress at a much slower pace and that include much more repetition and more hands-on, active participation at each stage of learning.

A national policy of differentiation attempts to ensure that all pupils are always working at the level that is just right for them. Differentiation means adjusting the work so that each pupil can learn. Schoolwork and homework can be differentiated in numerous ways — by level, by the amount a pupil is expected to do, by the time allowed, or by how the work is presented.

Effective differentiation is often not easy to implement. It can take a lot of the teacher's time and requires good organisation. The support available to organise differentiation effectively varies from school to school.

Differentiation solves some problems, but, like most solutions, it often creates a new set of problems. Some children feel embarrassed and demoralised when given obviously easier work. And sadly, even with conscientious differentiation, a significant minority of pupils are still left behind, not quite understanding, not quite remembering, and definitely not fulfilling their potential. Over time the gap in attainment among pupils in the same year continues to widen.

No teacher, no matter how gifted or dedicated, will ever care about a particular child's success as much as the parents of that child will. Most schools accept that in any given classroom most pupils will perform adequately, a few pupils (those commonly labelled 'quick, bright, able, gifted, highly intelligent') will excel, and a few pupils will continually struggle with learning.

A pupil who rarely experiences success will, over time, lose confidence and enthusiasm. He may begin to think of himself as a failure and a disappointment. Eventually he may even give up trying. So it is not at all surprising that these same pupils continue to scrape along the bottom, just getting by, year after year. No parents are happy for their child to be among the group of children who continue to feel unsuccessful.

Teachers may have a one-sided view of a child who is experiencing problems at school. They are not able to see all the areas, outside of school, where this child functions adequately or possibly even shines. Therefore, the teachers of a pupil who continually struggles with school learning may conclude that the child is in fact achieving his potential, but that unfortunately his potential is quite low.

Living with their child and seeing him in many different situations, parents are in a much better position to see his true potential. They are also in an ideal position to guide their child to do his best and be his best. These children need what schools often cannot provide:

- More individual instruction from an adult who understands about learning differences
- More time to take in and absorb the information they need to learn
- More frequent feedback, especially feedback about what they are doing right, so that they can build on their strengths
- More practice (including practice at evaluating their own work)
- A calmer, quieter, more orderly learning environment

The solution is not to waste time complaining or blaming the school, but to take charge and provide at home what your child needs but may not be getting from school. This book will explain how parents can do this using the daily homework time.

CHAPTER 4

WHY PARENTS NEED TO TAKE CHARGE OF THEIR CHILDREN'S EDUCATION, WHAT THIS REALLY MEANS, AND WHAT THIS CAN ACHIEVE

When pupils are taught the vital skills for school success, they are finally able, sometimes for the first time in their school lives, to fulfil their potential. They learn what they are capable of learning, and they apply what they have learned. Their curiosity, enthusiasm and self-confidence blossom, and they enjoy their 'job'. This is what parents want for their children. This is what every child deserves.

You may feel very strongly that your child's school should provide what he needs. Of course, that is true. You may want to do something to make that happen. You can work to help your school help your child more effectively. You can even make suggestions about how to improve the whole school system. But don't hold your breath waiting for systems to change. Reforms usually happen very slowly, and in the meantime your child may be missing out, possibly even suffering.

Instead of complaining or resigning yourself to an unsatisfactory situation, take action. You, the parent, can provide what your child needs in order to become a successful learner.

> Our children's education is far too important to leave up to the schools.

Knowing that there is something you can do will help you to feel positive, rather than discouraged, when your child encounters some of the inevitable problems associated with schooling.

Some parents decide to be the sole educators of their children, but that is not what most modern families choose to do. What I am suggesting is that parents see themselves as the most important educators of their children.

It is, of course, the teachers' responsibility to teach the school subjects. The parents' role, however, is just as important. Our job as parents is to prepare our child so that he or she can access and take advantage of everything the school has to offer. To achieve this we need to take on the responsibility for teaching and training the all-important skills for school success. This means:

- We will need to stay aware, day-by-day, of what is happening at school and how our child is responding.
- We will need to be advocates for our children, supporting them and working with the school (see box page 21).
- We will need to learn about and practise new ways of communicating with and guiding our children so that they become more and more cooperative, confident, motivated, self-reliant and considerate (see Section Two).
- We will need to closely supervise the daily homework time so that we establish productive, enjoyable homework habits (see Section Two).
- We will need to teach our child how to learn and how to do his best (see Section Three).
- We will need to fill in the gaps when the curriculum is moving too fast, leaving our child behind (see Section Four).

- Possibly most important of all, we will probably need to change the family's lifestyle in order to give each child the best possible chance to be, and feel, successful (see Chapter 9).

The above to-do list may seem quite daunting! You may be worried that you lack the patience or the education or the free time to take charge of your child's education. You will be pleased to learn that teaching the skills for school success does not require you to invest any more time supervising homework than you normally would. Instead, it asks you to use the Calmer, Easier, Happier Homework methods and to do things differently within the daily homework time.

You do not even need to remember much of what you learned at school because it is not your job to teach the subject matter your child should be learning at school. Your job will be to train your child in good habits and to break down indigestible lumps of learning into bite-sized 'micro-skills'. And as you put the Calmer, Easier, Happier Homework skills into practice, you will find that you need much less patience because you will encounter a lot less resistance or negativity and a lot more cooperation and enthusiasm.

KEY CONCEPT

Being an advocate for your child: Communicating effectively with the school

One important way that parents can help children to achieve their potential is to choose to see the school as a partner, not as an adversary. The following recommendations will help.

Put time and thought into building a positive relationship with your child's teachers long before any problems arise. This will smooth the way when you do need to address an uncomfortable situation. There are several ways to establish rapport with teachers, and I suggest you do them all:

- Whenever you see any of the teachers, even in passing, smile and greet them by name. This has the added benefit of influencing your child to like, trust and respect his teachers more.
- Frequently notice and mention to your children's teachers and to the head any aspects of the teaching or of the school's ethos that you are pleased about. If you cannot do this in person, you can send notes in to school every week. When parents are angry and are feeling powerless to affect how the school is dealing with their child, they may not feel able to focus on the positive. But the positive can always be found, if we make a decision to look for it.
- Attend as many school events as possible, not only the twice-yearly parents' evenings, but also the special evenings explaining aspects of the curriculum, the parents' association meetings and the fundraisers such as jumble sales and fêtes, etc. Think of this as an investment in your child's community.
- Mark all relevant school events on your calendar so that you do not forget about them or double-book yourself. Use a large family calendar that hangs at your child's eye level, and write these events in neatly so that your child can easily read them. He will see how seriously you take his education.
- Help in the classroom or around the school, volunteer to accompany school outings, help with fundraising or become a school governor. Even a working parent with a heavy

schedule can usually arrange to spare one hour each fortnight to contribute to the school community. Not only will
you learn a lot about the school, but you will also be in a
better position to influence practices and policies.

- Make a point of learning as much as you can, on an ongoing
  basis, about:
    - The teachers — their names, their strengths and weak-
      nesses, how they view the class, how they view your child
    - The curriculum
    - How progress is monitored
    - Methods of teaching
    - Methods of behaviour management, including rules,
      rewards and consequences
    - How teachers want homework to be dealt with at home

Homework and home learning are the keys to school success

The usual advice that parents are given about helping children
to do well at school is useful as far as it goes:

- Make sure that your child has a desk in a quiet, well-
  lighted area.
- Give him access to an appropriate dictionary and refer-
  ence materials.
- Show an interest.
- Make sure he sees you reading.
- Go to all parents' evenings.

Useful though this basic advice may be, it is not enough! Many
parents who have followed all these suggestions are still
worried because their children are not doing their best, either

at school or with their homework. Consequently, these children are not learning all that they could and should be learning, in terms of both school subjects and good habits.

The parents of these children and teenagers are frustrated and want to know what else they can do. Luckily, there are positive and effective alternatives to letting schoolwork and homework deteriorate until they become a huge source of friction in the family.

Homework is the one aspect of children's schooling that parents have the most access to and the most influence over. Therefore, it makes sense for parents to be proactive and to harness the huge potential of homework to improve academic learning and sensible work habits.

One could debate the relative merits of different types of homework, or even the value of homework per se, but that is not my brief. I want to help children and teens to feel successful. In schools where homework is set, most young people cannot be (or feel) successful unless they are handing their homework in on time and <u>doing their best</u> on their homework. And even when children are attending schools that do not set homework, I still always recommend that some formal academic home learning, targeted to the child's specific needs, be done daily.

I believe that regardless of ability or skill level, all children need to do homework because:

- All children have weak areas that need to be strengthened.
- All children should be stretched, and parents can do this better than teachers because parents know their child better and they can work one-to-one with that child.
- All children need to develop good work habits and become more and more self-reliant.

What is the Calmer, Easier, Happier Homework programme?

Who will do it?

The Calmer, Easier, Happier Homework programme requires your active participation six days a week, during term time and also during holidays. On days when you are not available, you will need to ask another adult to stand in.

What will you be doing?

Six days a week (including holidays) you will be closely supervising all your child's home learning: Homework, reading, memorising, revision and projects.

Where will you be doing this?

At home, or wherever you and your child happen to be during the *sacred homework time*, even in a hotel room if you are on holiday.

When will you do this?

Your participation will be needed for approximately one hour every day during the usual homework time. For younger children, the hour can be divided into two separate half-hours or even three sessions of twenty minutes each.

Why will you do this?

You need to take charge of your children's homework habits because these are the school success skills that will enhance learning, boost confidence and motivation, and enable your children to get the most from school and from all the other areas of their lives. Homework habits lead to school habits, which lead to life habits.

Most educators acknowledge that children forget a vast amount of what they learn at school. As adults, we generally have only a vague recollection of topics such as the Tudors, Ancient Egypt, the Greek gods, photosynthesis, strong and weak verbs, quadratic equations, etc. What most often remains, after we have forgotten many of the details of the subjects we studied, are the skills of literacy and numeracy, a great deal of 'general knowledge' and certain positive attitudes and mature habits, such as enthusiasm, perseverance, attention to detail and problem solving. These are some of the basic skills and habits that enable adults to be employable and to function adequately in many other areas of life, including relationships and leisure pursuits.

I am not suggesting that parents and teachers should focus solely on literacy and numeracy at the expense of history, science, geography, art, music, P.E., etc. Those subjects are intrinsically important for many reasons. And they can be exciting vehicles for the learning of literacy, numeracy and positive attitudes and habits.

How will you do this?

During the daily homework time you will establish routines and habits that will make homework productive and enjoyable.

In addition, there are often resources available within the school to help children who need something extra in order to access the curriculum. Parents need to inform themselves so that they can assess carefully, monitor thoroughly, liaise assertively yet diplomatically, and advocate relentlessly.

(You have noticed, I am sure, that so far I have been writing about your child as 'he' and 'him'. Throughout this book I will talk about both boys and girls, but most of my references will be to boys because boys make up more than three-quarters of all children who have problems with attention, learning and behaviour.)

• •

THE CALMER, EASIER, HAPPIER HOMEWORK RULES AND ROUTINES

CHAPTER 5

THE ESSENTIAL CALMER, EASIER, HAPPIER HOMEWORK RULES AND ROUTINES

My children are all teenagers now and homework is definitely calmer, easier and happier since we learned Noël's strategies, which was about five years ago.

Two of my kids had opposite problems from each other. The 12 year old was a typical boy, dashing through his work as if he just didn't care about it at all. My daughter, who was 14, spent hours every night getting her homework just right and getting herself exhausted. The solution, which we learned from Noël's book, was the same for both of them. We found out from their schools how much time the homework should take, and we made them stick to that. So my son had to do more and my daughter had to do less. For the first week they both complained. Then they got used to it. My son's work got better because he was paying more attention to it, and my daughter saw that when she had to, she could do good work in half the time. So we were able to spend time together as a family in the evenings. Of course, we started some other routines as well — no electronics until after homework, healthy snacks, practising micro-skills, lots more. My husband and I were worried that they'd hate the new rules, but they were happier, just like Noël said!

Mother of three teenagers

Only a very, very few children and teens have the maturity and motivation to create and maintain productive homework routines for themselves with no help from their parents.

Enjoyable, productive homework habits need to start out as rules that parents initially lay down as law. We must not expect our children to be happy about the new rules at first. But if we persevere, staying <u>friendly and firm,</u> over time, and sooner than you might think possible, resistance fades, the rules become accepted and even appreciated. The rules then gradually become routines, habits.

1. Have a sacred homework time every day (except Sundays)

Start the habit of having your child sit down and do homework, memorising or revision <u>every day</u>. Among other benefits, this is the way to train children and teenagers in the habit of revising well in advance of tests, rather than cramming for one or two nights before a test.

> Why is it so important to establish a daily homework schedule for your child and to make sure that he sticks to it?
> Because <u>routines reduce resistance.</u>

A routine that parents insist upon is a force external to the child. The routine frees the child's mind from two very negative, debilitating emotions:

- The nagging worry (often called 'pressure' or 'stress') about when, or even if, he will be able to force himself to start his homework
- The guilt he feels when he leaves his homework too late to do a good job or when he manages to avoid it altogether

This combination of anxiety and guilt is very destructive.

If your child is not yet in the habit of doing some homework every day, you may need to start with short daily sessions. And of course you will need to make sure that the work is just challenging enough that he experiences satisfaction rather than frustration.

Do not skip weekends

Two or more days in a row without homework can make re-establishing the homework routines on Monday evening that much more difficult. A break of two days is a long time in the life of a child or teenager. During this time he can mentally start sliding out of the productive habits that you have been putting so much effort into reinforcing during the week.

One day off a week is the optimum. One day off will be greatly appreciated, and it will not undermine the weekly routines. It is wise to designate Sunday as the homework-free day, which means that all weekend homework and revision need to be completed on Saturday. Your child will have the gift of one day a week when no thought of work need enter his mind. This is especially important for the pupil who is not feeling successful.

Wherever possible, plan for homework to be done at the same time every day

That way it is predictable, and therefore easier, for everyone to remember and accept. Of course, this may not always be possible because modern life has so many variables: after-school activities, parents' work schedules, household tasks, emergencies, etc. But you can still establish routines. Homework can be at the same time every Monday, even if on Tuesdays it has to be at a different time and on Wednesdays at yet another time. Make a chart and post it in a prominent place. Refer to it frequently. This will greatly reduce confusion and resistance. Making homework an absolutely clear priority by devoting <u>some</u> time to it every day is an important key to school success.

KEY CONCEPT

What to do during the daily homework time if the school has not set any homework that is due the following day?

- Have your child get a head start on homework that is due in a few days, rather than allowing him to leave it until the evening before it is due.
- Have him do some revision of a topic that is causing him trouble or some practising of a micro-skill you think he needs to improve. Some examples of micro-skills might be: reading aloud with expression, practising last week's or last term's spelling words, practising handwriting or punctuation or multiplication facts. Even in secondary school, these, and similar micro-skills, may still need to be improved (see Chapter 11 for a discussion of micro-skills).

2. Establish how long homework should take

For most children, I would expect to gradually work up to <u>one or two hours of homework every evening</u>, depending on the school's guidelines. One hour is usually the minimum time needed in primary school and two hours in senior school to:

- Do a thorough, careful job on homework
- Read to a parent
- Work a bit every day on special reports, projects or coursework
- Revise well in advance for quizzes, tests and exams
- Practise a few micro-skills in order to improve weak areas

You will need to find out from your child's school what the guidelines are in each year for how long homework should take. The school may say something like: Two subjects each weeknight and three over the weekend, each to take approximately half an hour. However long the school says that the homework should take, <u>do not let your child spend longer than the recommended amount of time on it</u>. This rule is important for a number of reasons:

- The child who wastes time earlier in the evening by complaining or arguing may panic a few hours later and plead to be allowed to stay up past his bedtime to finish. This child may end up with no guilt-free leisure time. He is left with the feeling that all he ever does is schoolwork and homework, even though we know that for a large chunk of his evening he was staring sullenly at, rather than actually doing, his homework.
- Some children, particularly those who are sensitive or unconfident, become perfectionists and would choose, if allowed, to spend most of their evening working. This is no good for them; all children need to have 'downtime' every day.

● A child may be working diligently, but find the work so difficult that it takes him longer to finish than it should. He too needs guilt-free leisure time. And the school needs to know that he is not capable of completing the homework within the suggested time. Otherwise, the teachers will continue to set homework that is not appropriate for this child.

State schools are required by law to differentiate the delivery of the curriculum to enable all pupils to learn. The child who spends all evening working should not simply be given less homework. Each of his teachers will need to find out where the difficulty lies and then teach him from that point, rather than expecting him to understand something that he does not yet understand.

When a child attends a highly academic, prestigious school and is just managing to hang in there by spending an inordinate amount of time on homework and revision (and possibly extra tutoring), the parents may be reluctant to reveal the truth to the school. They may worry that the school would conclude that a child who is struggling so much does not belong there. And the school may be right. This can be a blow to parents, and even to the child, who may blame himself for letting his parents down. When parents are positive and learn to adjust their expectations more realistically, the child will follow suit and take in his stride the move to a more suitable school, if necessary.

We should also not let children spend <u>less</u> time on their homework than the school's guidelines. We need to guide children into the habit of doing their best, which always entails slowing down and focusing on accuracy, thoroughness and excellent presentation. Otherwise they will develop the habit of rushing through their work to get it over with quickly, and will not be learning what we want them to be learning. Occasionally a child's homework is so easy for him that, even with good attention to detail, it doesn't take him the full amount of time the school recommends. If this happens a lot, ask his teacher to give him more challenging work. If the teacher is too busy to do that, you will need to do that yourself.

KEY CONCEPT

Eliminate distractions

There should be no distractions in the whole house during the sacred homework time. You, the parent, need to be in charge of eliminating all temptations in order to make it easier for your child to concentrate. It is the parent's job to remove all potential distractions, rather than nagging about them. Before the home-work even comes out of the school bag:

- Make sure that no screen is on within the child's earshot.
- Put the telephone on answerphone and turn down the ringer.
- Together with your child, remove all toys and unnecessary equipment from the table.
- Put any pets that might distract in another room.
- If you have a toddler who cannot safely be left in another room, set him up with a highly absorbing activity (one that you bring out only at this time) so that he will be learning not to interrupt the older sibling's homework session.

3. Work before play

One of the best ways to help children take homework seriously is to make, and then enforce, the rule that homework and revision need to be completed, to <u>the parents' satisfaction,</u> before leisure activities can begin, for example:

- Television, social media, computer games, etc.
- Telephoning or texting friends
- Going out
- Playing music, etc.

This rule helps ease children into the habit of <u>earning</u> the goodies in life, rather than <u>expecting</u> instant gratification.

After school, most children need to unwind and have something to eat before they plunge into their homework. A healthy snack and an <u>active break</u> will relax and refresh them: a short bike ride, playing catch, trampolining, etc. Sitting in front of a screen, however, does not refresh or motivate; in fact, it saps enthusiasm for any other activity. Remember that people managed to relax without the help of screens from the dawn of time until about fifty years ago!

4. Divide each homework task into three stages

This teaches children and teenagers the habit of paying attention to detail and doing their best. Here are the three stages:

Stage One: The *think-through* (See Chapter 6 for an explanation of *think-throughs*)
Stage Two: Your child works on her own
Stage Three: The improving stage

Stage One: The parent and the child do a think-through

In this vital first stage, we help bring back into the child's working memory whatever he needs to keep in mind in order to do the task well so that he can learn what there is to learn from the task. We do this by questioning, which is far more effective than telling. Even for simple pieces of work, have him tell you <u>exactly</u> what he needs to do and how and why. Ask leading questions to guide him to think carefully about aspects of the task that he may be unaware of or may wish to ignore:

How many pages does this essay have to be?

What will you do if you can't spell a word?

Does your teacher expect you to write full sentences or one-word answers?

Where do you put the carry number?

The parent's job is to ask the questions; the child's job is to think for himself and to answer the parent's questions. The only time that you will switch from asking him to telling him what to do and how to do it is when one of his answers is incorrect, incomplete or confused. Once the point has been clarified to your satisfaction, ask him the same question again, as many times as necessary, until he can tell you exactly what he needs to do and how he will do it. For more about *think-throughs*, see Chapter 6.

Stage Two: The child does the homework, without any help

Homework is designed to be done by the child, not by the parent. With very few exceptions, homework is not meant to be a collaborative effort! Homework should be ongoing training in self-reliance, so in the second stage the child works completely on his own, <u>with no help</u>. If you think he might need help with some aspect of his homework, include questions about that in the Stage One *think-through*.

Once Stage Two begins, your child is on his own. A thorough *think-through* in Stage One will eliminate many of the mistakes he usually makes, but of course he will still make some mistakes. When your child makes a mistake during Stage Two, do not say a word; do not frown, nudge, shake your head or point to the mistake.

Until your child is more mature and more motivated, I recommend that you stay in the room during Stage Two, so that you can Descriptively Praise and Reflectively Listen every few minutes, if necessary (see Chapter 5). But don't answer any questions or even give clues. Stage Two is the child's job.

Stage Three: The last stage is the improving stage

This is the time when we comment on what the child has produced. Together, the parent and the child evaluate the work, and then the child makes the improvements. It often helps to leave a period of time between the composing in Stage Two and the evaluating in Stage Three. This enables the child's brain to transition from one function to the other.

1 **First, each of you finds three good (or at least OK) things to Descriptively Praise about the piece of work.** You must not rush this part of Stage Three. Children learn

a great deal from thinking about what they have done <u>right</u>. Don't let your child say vaguely, 'It's OK,' or even, 'My answers are right,' which is a bit more descriptive. Instead, insist that she be specific. She could say, 'I wrote four facts about photo-synthesis,' or, 'I looked up how to spell Mediterranean, so I know it's right'.

2 **Then, you and your child each notice and mention two things about that piece of work that your child will need to improve.** The more thoroughly you have done the *think-through* in Stage One, the less there will be that needs correcting or improving in Stage Three. Even so, on most days you will probably notice more than two things that could be improved. But mention only two; otherwise you risk discouraging your child. Rather than telling him what his mistake was, give a *diagnostic response*. This will teach him, over time, how to solve homework problems on his own. Let's say he has written '10' as the answer to '5 x 5 = ?'. You can say, '10 would be the answer if you were adding'. Then wait while his brain figures out what he should do.

Stage Three is very important, so give it plenty of time. And don't be surprised if your child resists noticing and acknowledging his good work as well as his mistakes. He may be in the habit of thinking his homework is over as soon as he stops writing. Your insistence on Stage Three may come as a shock at first.

5. Do not let your child leave the hardest task until last

Make sure your child tackles the most troublesome subjects or tasks while his brain is freshest. This will promote optimum learning. It will also remove the nagging dread that eats away at anyone's good humour when they are putting off something that they expect will be unpleasant.

KEY CONCEPT

Build in realistic breaks

Learning can be frustrating and emotionally exhausting for children and teens who are not yet successful learners. To prevent overload, insist that your child has an active break (not in front of a screen) every fifteen to thirty minutes, depending on his age and on his current ability to concentrate on homework. Decide in advance when your child can have breaks. This will, over time, curb the child's tendency to complain or to invent ingenious excuses for getting up and doing something else.

6. Make use of the holidays

Holidays are a perfect time to improve school success skills — painlessly! You may have heard of the 'summer slide'. This refers to how much academic ground children lose over the six weeks of the summer holidays. At best they may lose just a couple of months, but with pupils who are finding school difficult, it can be a loss of almost a year's worth of skills. But the summer slide is not inevitable. Just half an hour a day of academic work during the holidays can keep your child's brain oiled, so it doesn't get rusty and seize up.

Don't leave it up to your child or teen to discipline herself about holiday homework, reading, projects or revision. Even with the best intentions, she is likely to put it off. The holidays seem so long; it feels to her as if she will have plenty of time to tackle it next week . . . or the week after . . . or the week after. And then, before you know it, the end of the holiday is in sight and panic sets in. This doesn't help children to do their best.

Even before the holidays begin, sit down with your child and together plan how much needs to be done, each week and each day, in order to finish all the holiday homework or revising with one full week to spare (in case there is a hiccup and you find that some bit of it takes much longer than you both had anticipated).

- The best time for the half-hour of academic work is after breakfast and before fun. That way you all know that it is done and out of the way before the day begins. And whatever else your children do that day, it will feel like more of a treat because they have already done that half-hour of homework.
- If no homework has been set for the holidays, help each child start a project on something that interests them, such as dinosaurs, football or the Olympics. Work on it together six days a week. Remember to Descriptively Praise (see Chapter 6) sensible work habits and be enthusiastic (even if you don't feel like it!)
- To establish the habit of reading for pleasure, set aside ten to twenty minutes each day when the whole family sits together in the same room, each silently reading from a book of their choice. Even a child who thinks he hates reading can cope with this short amount of time. And day by day, you will be strengthening his stamina and reducing his resistance to reading.

Identify three micro-skills your child needs to improve and help her to revise each one for five minutes a day. You will be surprised how much progress she makes in just a few weeks. (See Chapter 11 for more on micro-skills.)

KEY CONCEPT

Train your child to be organised

Disorganisation is very distracting. Do not expect an immature or impulsive or resistant child to know how to organise himself. You will need to train him. Allow on the table at any given time only what the child needs for that step of that task. Do not put his other work away yourself; that is your child's job. Do not tell him where to put things; thinking about that is also his job. Instead, Prepare for Success by asking leading questions:

Where do you want to put your diagram so it won't get wrinkled?

Where should you put the highlighter so that you'll know where it is the next time you need it?

How will you keep this section of your project separate from the other section?

Your child may respond to these questions by taking a sensible action, for example by putting the highlighter back in his pencil case. In addition to action, require him to answer your questions in words. This will help the overarching principles of organisation to sink in to his long-term memory.

CHAPTER 6

ESTABLISHING AND REINFORCING THE NEW HOMEWORK RULES AND ROUTINES

I'm a foster parent, and earlier this year I had a very difficult foster child living with me for a few months. He was nine, and before he came to live with me he had never had to do any homework at all. So you can imagine what it was like trying to get him to do it. I was just getting crosser and crosser until a colleague told me about Calmer, Easier, Happier Homework. Descriptive Praise was so helpful! I started doing lots of think-throughs, about ten every day, which is what Noël recommends when there's a lot of resistance. I was asking James questions like 'When it's homework time, where should you be sitting?' 'When I say it's homework time, what should you do?' 'When can you get up?' 'What will your reward be when you finish all your homework? In a few days he started doing his homework without tantrums or whingeing! But I made the mistake of forgetting about the think-throughs once he stopped making such a fuss about home-work, and he just slid right back to refusing. So I realised I had to do the think-throughs for much, much longer. But it was well worth it. I also did lots of Descriptive Praise. And it wasn't just homework that got better. He became so sweet and polite. Now I use these techniques with all my foster kids.

Foster parent of one child, aged 9

By now you may be wondering how you will ever make the new rules and routines you decided on in Chapter 5 stick, and how you are going to apply them to your specific situation. In this chapter I will show that this can be easier than you think if you follow the Calmer, Easier, Happier Parenting strategies.

Consistency is key

Consistent routines and rules help children and teens to feel comfortable because their environment is predictable and therefore emotionally safe.

A parent may not want to live with consistent routines and rules because they are as binding on the parent as they are on the child. Consistency limits our freedom to be spontaneous. But consistency is what children need. This especially applies to the more sensitive, intense or emotionally immature child, whose natural rhythms are often quite inconsistent. He needs our help to get and stay on an even keel. The child who is constantly wangling for an exception is the very child who cannot handle exceptions well. He gets hooked on trying to get away with minor or major misbehaviour. He stores the inconsistencies in his long-term memory and uses them as ammunition to try and get us to change our minds the next time.

The more easy-going, laid-back child is better able to deal with some exceptions and changes to the established routines. He takes these in his stride. But a lack of clarity and consistency adversely affects even the relatively easy child. He too can become an arch manipulator if parents say one thing and do another.

When routines and rules are not consistent, far too much of a child's energies go into testing, arguing, wheedling for exceptions and splitting hairs. Paradoxically, consistent rules and routines free children by allowing them to put more thought and energy into their primary developmental task, which is learning in its broadest sense: noticing, experimenting, making inferences, drawing conclusions and applying to new situations the knowledge they have gained.

Consistency has the added benefit of depersonalising parental requirements. The child can see that the parent is not making up a rule on the spur of the moment out of anger or anxiety. The child learns to accept even an unwelcome restriction with a rather philosophical attitude of, 'Oh well, this is the way life is,' almost as if the rule were a force of nature, beyond anyone's control.

The Calmer, Easier, Happier Parenting strategies

There are a number of very powerful Calmer, Easier, Happier Parenting strategies that parents can use to help children and teenagers overcome their understandable resistance to the new homework rules and routines.

Preparing for Success

Preparing for Success includes a number of techniques that lead to more enjoyable and productive homework habits and to children achieving their potential.

Becoming a United Front (consistency between parents)

One of the contributing factors for ongoing homework problems is children seeing that parents do not agree about the rules and routines or do not *follow through* in the same way.

Often parents assume that becoming united would be very difficult or even impossible. There is a tendency for parents to let this very important type of consistency slide because they may feel that trying to get united would just lead to arguments. It doesn't have to.

Parents need to set aside a chunk of time, perhaps half an hour, with no children around and with no distractions.
Together, talk about which of the Calmer, Easier, Happier Homework rules and routines you want to establish, even if you cannot quite believe that you could ever make them happen consistently.

Where necessary, compromise for a United Front. And no criticising of your partner's ideas! Working together also makes it much harder for children to divide and conquer with complaints such as 'But Dad said I didn't have to'.

If you are a single parent, do this step with a friend because two heads are better than one. Once you know how you want the homework routines and rules to work, write them down, in as much detail as possible: who, what, when, where, why and how.

Clear rules and expectations

Clarifying the routines and rules, in and of itself, can prevent many (but not all) flare-ups of resistance or misbehaviour.

1   **In addition to the Calmer, Easier, Happier Homework rules and routines, have a few overarching rules that will cover many different situations.**
    I suggest the following all-purpose rules for children and teens:

- Do what you are told, the first time and without a fuss. (This covers what you want your children to start doing as well as what you want them to stop doing.)
- Instead of interrupting a parent who is talking or concentrating on something, say 'Excuse me' and then wait for the parent to stop talking and to look at you. (We should set a good example by doing the same.)
- Instead of complaining, make a polite request.

2 **Now make up and write down some rules and routines for yourself to follow.**
These will improve cooperation much faster than any rules we make for our children! For example, a powerful rule for parents is: As soon as you find that you are getting annoyed with your children, immediately switch into Descriptive Praise mode (later in this chapter I explain how Descriptive Praise works). This will usually gain you cooperation more quickly than any other tactic.

3 **At a neutral time, both parents sit down with one child to tell her the new homework rules or routines.**
Talking to each child separately enables you to tailor the rules for each. Also, the possibly mocking or obstructive attitude of one child will not influence the other siblings.
Before you start talking, emphasise that this meeting will last no more than ten minutes and set a timer to make sure that you stop exactly on time. An angry, suspicious or resistant child will be able to accept and participate in such a discussion more willingly when he knows that the ordeal he anticipates will soon be over. Ten minutes will probably not be enough time to explain all the rules and routines you want to see happening. You will need to have additional ten-minute meetings daily until you are satisfied

that everyone in the family understands and remembers all the homework routines and rules. You will know they understand when they can tell you.

Open the discussion by explaining (in a calm, friendly, assertive voice, taking care not to sound either tentative or irritated) that parents as well as children have responsibilities about homework. Draw a line down the centre of a blank piece of paper and label the two sides something like: 'Mum and Dad need to' and 'Henry needs to'. Instead of telling your child what the new homework routines and rules will be, ask each person in turn, starting with the child, to say some of the homework responsibilities that he can think of, whether yours or his own. If you like, you can call them policies or guidelines, rather than rules. This may make them more palatable, especially for teenagers.

You will be pleasantly surprised to discover that your child knows most of the routines and rules, even those that he regularly ignores or continually tries to negotiate about. Write down neatly in the correct columns any that you agree with, refraining from making any comments that your child might perceive as negative.

One parent reported that her son replied, 'Mum, write down on your side that you should stay out of it. The school says it's our responsibility. We're old enough'. This mother bit her tongue and managed not to retort with a snappy one-liner, such as, 'I'll be glad to stay out of it when you can prove to me that you're doing it properly'. Instead, she took a deep breath to calm herself and said, with a smile, 'My job is to help you get into good habits. So I can't stay out of it just yet because you still need help with some of your habits, like starting early enough. But maybe pretty soon I'll be able to. We would both like that'. By pausing and collecting her thoughts before she spoke, this mother conveyed the same information, but in a much more positive, less blaming way.

KEY CONCEPT

Refer to this list of rules every day

Use the list of rules that you and your children have generated as an aide-memoire during the daily homework sessions. This list will remind you of the many things that your child is not doing wrong at any given moment. Because you have taken the time to clarify and explain what you want, you will find that there is now much more that you can Descriptively Praise. Later in the chapter I will explain about Descriptive Praise, a particular way of appreciating our children that is highly motivating. The more our children hear about their OK behaviour, the more of it we will see.

Using think-throughs to help your child remember the rules and routines

In Chapter 5 I explained about the three stages of homework. The first stage is the *think-through. Think-throughs* are an alternative to repeating, reminding, lecturing and telling off, which are not effective at improving habits. For rapid progress, do *think-throughs* about homework at many other times of the day, not just during the homework session.

The hallmarks of a *think-through* are:

- Each *think-through* takes only one minute (except for Stage One *think-throughs*, which may take up to five minutes).
- *Think-throughs* happen only at neutral times, by which I

mean times when neither the parent nor the child is upset, in a rush or in front of a screen.

- *Think-throughs* are always about what your child should do in the future, not about what she did wrong in the past.
- A *think-through* is used for introducing a new rule or for clarifying an old rule that has been neglected because of inconsistent *follow through*.
- Whenever possible, do *think-throughs* with both parents. This will show your child that the rule is important. And everyone will know that everyone knows the rule. This eliminates a lot of manipulating and trying to divide and conquer.
- The parents ask leading questions, and the child has to answer sensibly and politely.
- Do the *think-throughs* with one child at a time, even if the same rule applies to more than one child. The effectiveness of *think-throughs* comes from the child answering the parents' questions. With two children, even if one is answering the question, the other isn't.

Let's say that you would like to establish a new rule that your child shows you his homework each evening after it is completed. In the *think-through,* once you've stated the new rule, you can ask questions such as:

What's the new rule?

When is the new routine going to start?

Where will we both be sitting when you show me your completed homework?

Who do you need to show your homework to every night?

When do you need to show us your homework?

You can expect children and teens who don't yet feel good about their homework to resist answering the *think-through* questions at first. They may roll their eyes or answer 'I don't know,' or mumble. They may give you a jokey answer, look away or even state categorically that they will not answer. Don't panic. There is nothing inherently awful about children being required to answer questions of this type! Children answer their teachers' questions every day, even when they don't feel like it. The mostly likely reason for any negative reaction is that the child can see that the parents are getting back in charge. So persevere.

In this next example, a teenager was regularly being disrespectful to her parents during homework time. Some of the *think-through* questions her parents asked her at a neutral time were:

When you're feeling annoyed, what can you say instead of saying the homework is stupid?

What's a respectful way to answer when Mum or Dad tell you to do something?

How can you show us you're upset without being rude?

You may find this hard to believe, but answering the *think-through* questions helps children and teens to get into more mature, more sensible habits. This is because as the child is telling you the answer to the *think-through* questions, he is visualising himself doing it right. The more often you do these one-minute *think-throughs*, the more often your child will be visualising himself doing the right thing, and the sooner those positive images will be transferred into his long-term memory, where they influence behaviour quite quickly.

You may have many questions about this new strategy. In *Calmer, Easier, Happier Parenting* I address all the questions and concerns parents have about *think-throughs*.

KEY CONCEPT

Don't rush homework — build in extra time instead

Remember that a child's tempo is different from an adult's. When children don't feel like doing something, they're often lethargic and distractible. If we rush our children, trying to get them to do what we want faster than is comfortable for them, misbehaviour of one sort or another will result. They may ignore us, dawdle, come up with excuses or dig their heels in and simply refuse. So to make it more likely that a child will cooperate, we need to build some extra time into every part of a child's routine. This may not feel easy, but it's much easier than dealing with the resistance that occurs when we're hurrying our children.

Scheduling frequent Special Time to enhance motivation

A great deal of misbehaviour, negative attention seeking and complaining about homework can be eliminated by giving children and teens the positive attention they crave, need and deserve. As you will see, Descriptive Praise is one important and easy way to give children this positive attention.

Another important way is for the parent to arrange to have Special Time with each child — one-on-one with no siblings in sight, no screen on in the background, no checking your mobile phone and no distractions. Special Time has many benefits. One is that we see our child's best side when he is not interacting with a sibling, and our child sees our best side when we are not focused on getting something done. Special Time builds a very strong bond between parent and child, and this bond can stand us in very good stead when a child is reluctant to do her homework. She will want to please us more because Special Time awakens in children the desire to make parents proud.

If the idea of daily Special Time appeals to you but seems impossible to achieve, be willing to start with very small chunks of time, for example ten or fifteen minutes a day. You will soon come to enjoy the Special Time with each child separately; you will look forward to it and feel nourished by it. You will soon find yourself planning much longer chunks of Special Time alone with each child at weekends and holidays.

Get into the habit of spending your Special Time together in ways that do not cost money; card games, board games, puzzles, Lego, drawing, crafts, making a meal together, throwing and catching a Frisbee (easier for a young or uncoordinated child to handle than a ball), going for walks, DIY, having a picnic tea in the park, exploring in the garden.

At first, self-conscious teens and preteens will probably turn up their noses at most of these 'uncool' activities, so you need to persevere. Otherwise you could easily get sucked into regularly taking them to the cinema, shopping or out for a meal for their Special Time. All those activities cost money and often require planning and driving, and they can result in your feeling resentful and martyred when the child does not appreciate the trouble you have taken or the expense.

Frequent, predictable Special Time benefits all family members. The child's self-confidence, his enthusiasm for life, his willingness to tackle uncomfortable tasks and his motivation to please his parents all grow steadily when the most important people in his world are demonstrating an ongoing desire to spend time just with him. For both parents and child, this Special Time results in many pleasant memories, and these make it easier during any confrontation for the parent to remember the child's good qualities and for the child to remember the parent's good qualities. Everyone stays calmer.

In *Calmer, Easier, Happier Parenting* I give many more ideas for how a busy parent can manage to have Special Time alone with each child.

Following through

Following through is a term that refers to how we respond to cooperation or to its opposite. When we think about *following through*, our minds usually jump automatically to consequences for misbehaviour. But I want to start by discussing how we can effectively *follow through* when the child has cooperated or has remembered the rules and routines. We need to regularly *follow through* after good behaviour because that is the most effective method of reinforcing cooperation, motivation and self-reliance. But it is easy to overlook good behaviour. When a child is doing the right thing, we often grab the opportunity to turn our attention to the next task on our to-do list.

Even a child who is frequently resistant about homework will occasionally do what you say the first time you say it. He might open his exercise book without being told, he might remember to underline the title of his essay, or he might answer you politely. Often parents take these positive behaviours for granted because they believe that this level of cooperation is no more than they have a right to expect from the child. This is an understandable reaction, but it is short-sighted. Until your child is cooperative, motivated and self-reliant <u>most of the time</u>, we cannot simply assume that he will be. We need to reinforce the little bits of positive behaviour in order to get more positive behaviour. Parents report that they sometimes hesitate to point out what their child has done right, in case that reminds her that she could be acting up. That does happen occasionally, of course, especially with a very impulsive child and especially in the early weeks of this new plan. But that is not a good enough reason to refrain from *following through* for positive behaviour.

Descriptive Praise

Descriptive Praise is a strategy you can use many, many times every day. The more you Descriptively Praise, the sooner the new, more positive homework habits will be established.

The type of praise we generally give our children is full of superlatives: 'Well done!' 'Good boy!' 'You're so clever!' 'That's brilliant!'

We often praise with superlatives like this because we want to help our children feel confident or we want to encourage them to keep trying when they're finding something difficult or scary. One problem with this over-the-top praise is that our children do not believe us. They can see that the rest of the world doesn't think they are amazingly wonderful. Therefore they conclude one of two things: Either that we do not really believe that they are terrifically clever and talented but are exaggerating to try and make them feel good, or that we do believe all the superlatives simply because we love them.

Descriptive Praise, however, is a very different kind of praise. It is a very powerful motivator because it helps children want to please us and because it gives them very detailed information about what they can do to please us. Descriptive

Praise consists of leaving out the superlatives, and instead, making a point of noticing and mentioning every tiny step in the right direction:

- Small improvements in behaviour, attitude, homework habits, attention to detail, social skills, etc.
- Behaviour or work that is not wonderful or terrific, but just OK (actions that you might ordinarily take for granted)
- The absence of negative behaviour

At first when you start using Descriptive Praise, you may worry that your children will not realise you are praising them if you don't tack on 'well done' or 'that's fantastic' at the end of your sentence. In fact, they will know they are being praised because you will be talking about what they did right, your face will look pleased and your tone of voice will sound pleased.

Descriptive Praise is so motivating because it taps into a universal truth about humans: all of us (even children, even teenagers) are disposed to want to please the people who are pleasant to us. When I talk about being pleasant to our children, I do not mean indulging them or giving in; I mean showing our appreciation and approval, being friendly and polite. In addition, all children desperately want their parents to be proud of them. With Descriptive Praise, even those children and teenagers who had given up trying to please their parents quite soon start to feel better and behave better.

Here are some examples of Descriptive Praises that can motivate a reluctant child or teenager to accept the new homework rules and routines. Each Descriptive Praise takes only a few seconds to utter:

Following instructions
You did exactly what I told you to do.

You took your books out as soon as I asked. No time-wasting!

Thanks for not arguing.

Following routines and rules
You're following the new essay plan, and you didn't need any reminders. That shows maturity.

You told yourself the right thing to do, and then you did it. That's self-reliance.

You're remembering the new rule.

You're still writing, even though that noise might be disturbing.

Staying on task
Instead of giving up when it felt hard, you re-read the instructions. Very sensible.

I see you've been sitting for ten minutes, without once getting up.

You've stopped tapping the table. It's much more peaceful now.

Paying attention to details
You noticed your own mistake. And you're correcting it without my having to tell you to.

You've written four sentences, and three of them start with a capital letter. You're mostly remembering the rule.

I told you to write your answers in full sentences, and you did, even though it takes longer.

Every letter in this word is sitting exactly on the line.

There's no clutter on this desk.

Politeness and consideration
You're waiting patiently.

You're using your indoor voice now.

I appreciate that you didn't interrupt me.

Thanks for looking at me while I'm talking to you.

You might be feeling annoyed, but all I hear are polite words.

Positive attitudes
You weren't sure how to answer that comprehension question, but you had a go. That was brave.

You didn't say 'I don't know'. You took a sensible guess.

You're not complaining.

When we frequently show that we are pleased, our children see that they can please us. The more we notice and mention their positive behaviour, attitudes and work habits, the more cooperative, motivated and self-reliant our children and teens will become.

I challenge you to start with ten Descriptive Praises per day per child. You will find that it feels so good (for the parent as well as for the child) and is so motivating that soon you will be Descriptively Praising easily ten times each hour.

Never Ask Twice

When we are teaching and training more mature homework habits, there will be many times when we want to tell our child what to do or how to do something. These are called 'start behaviours'. There will, of course, also be times when we want our child to stop doing something, and those are called 'stop behaviours'. This next strategy, Never Ask Twice, is specifically for 'start behaviours'.

When we ask a child to do something with her homework and she doesn't cooperate straightaway, it's tempting to ask again . . . and again . . . and again. But the more we repeat ourselves, the less our children are motivated to listen. There is an alternative to repeating and reminding and nagging and cajoling and threatening and eventually shouting. There is a way to get children into the habit of taking us seriously and doing what we ask the first time we ask. The strategy that achieves this is called the Never Ask Twice method. You'll find that when you commit to using the Never Ask Twice method for all 'start behaviours', you won't be feeling nearly so frustrated.

Never Ask Twice has six steps. Most of the time you will only need the first three steps to achieve cooperation, but the remaining three steps are there for the times when your child is particularly resistant.

Step One: Stop what you are doing and go to your child. Stand in front of him and look at him.

In this step you are not yet speaking. Step One may be the hardest step of all; it may feel almost impossible in the middle of a busy day to take the time to stop everything. Instead, we tend to give instructions when we're not looking at the child and the child is not looking at us. We may not even be in the same room.

Standing is an important part of this step because standing shows that you are serious. Standing is very powerful. It conveys that you're in charge, that you know what you want and that you expect it to happen. (If you use these new strategies consistently, the time will come when you won't have to be standing in order to be taken seriously, but for now you probably do.)

Step Two: Wait for your child to stop what he's doing and look up at you.

He may be sitting in front of his open exercise book scowling mutinously. He may be playing with his ruler. Wait until he puts down whatever is in his hand and looks up at you. You might think he will never look up, but he will.

You can help your child want to look at you by Descriptively Praising something he is doing that is OK. Remember that the Never Ask Twice strategy is for 'start behaviours' so your child won't be doing anything wrong at that moment. You simply want him to start doing the next thing. If you've been taking my previous advice and doing lots of Descriptive Praise, your child will want to look at you.

Step Three: Now it is time to tell your child what you want him to do — clearly, simply and only once.

You might say:

Show me your history homework, please.
Now it's time to do a think-through about your geography quiz.

Open your book at the right page, please.

Once again, this may be hard to believe, but if you've done Steps One and Two, by the time you get to Step Three most children, most of the time, will do what you ask. You're speaking in a friendly, firm and respectful way, and children will usually respond with cooperation. The more you can discipline yourself to use the Never Ask Twice method for all 'start behaviours' (outside of homework sessions as well), the sooner you will find that your children will cooperate after Step Three. But in case your child is feeling particularly rebellious that day, we have three more steps.

Step Four: Ask your child to tell you what he's supposed to do.

This usually gets cooperation. At first you may find that your child is complaining or possibly even insulting you as he does what you have asked. Refrain from telling him off, and focus on the fact that he did what he was asked to do even though he didn't want to. After he has calmed down and is no longer upset, have him do an *action replay* (see Consequences, later in this chapter). But in case Step Four has not yet resulted in cooperation, go on to Step Five.

Step Five: Stand and wait, without arguing, without justifying, without getting sidetracked.

Don't repeat yourself. Just stand and wait. That is usually enough to get your child to take you seriously and to do what he's supposed to do. But just in case this is a really bad day, go to Step Six.

Step Six: While you are standing and waiting, Descriptively Praise any steps in the right direction and Reflectively Listen to how your child might be feeling.

These are some Descriptive Praises you might say:

You've picked up your pencil.

You've taken your book out of your bag.

You're not crying now.

Reflective Listening (which I talk more about next) is about imagining how your child might be feeling:

Maybe you're worried I'll be cross if you make a mistake.

You're probably angry that I'm saying it's time to start your essay now.

Maybe you're not sure what to write.

Descriptive Praise and Reflective Listening both help soften a child's resistance. If you're willing to do these Six Steps, your child will cooperate. If he's in the habit of having tantrums, then it's possible that during the first week or so of using these new strategies he may cry or scream or swear or throw himself about or storm off. A child who is likely to have a tantrum over homework is usually also prone to tantrums at other times of day, for example, mealtimes, getting ready in the morning and bedtimes. Tantrums can be very upsetting for parents and sometimes even frightening. Once again, I'd like to refer you to *Calmer, Easier, Happier Parenting*, where I explain in detail how to minimise and prevent tantrums.

Reflective Listening

Now let's talk about what to do when children are <u>not</u> doing what we want them to do. You may be assuming that this is where consequences come in, but in fact there is another strategy, called Reflective Listening, that I want to talk about first because it is far more effective than most consequences at motivating children to do the right thing.

Reflective Listening motivates children and overcomes resistance by helping them to see the parent as an ally rather than as the enemy. It also repairs damage to self-esteem and self-confidence. Reflective Listening is not always an easy skill for parents to master, but it is very effective. You will find yourself using this technique many times every day, whenever your children are upset, whether about homework or about anything else.

The benefits of Reflective Listening are that it helps an angry or anxious child to feel heard and understood. This can defuse uncomfortable emotions and potentially explosive situations. The child starts to relax and no longer feels that he needs to act up in order to make a point or to get the parents' attention. Once he feels heard, he often automatically turns his attention towards problem solving. Over time, Reflective Listening teaches children and teenagers a vocabulary for expressing their feelings in words rather than through tantrums, whingeing or misbehaviour. Reflective Listening has four steps:

Step One: You consciously make a point of setting aside your completely understandable feelings of frustration, guilt, confusion or despair.

This is not always easy to achieve, but it becomes much easier when we make a point of remembering that it is not the child's fault that he is misbehaving or being resistant. He has drifted into negative homework habits, often because his difficulties have not yet been properly addressed. 'Fault' is a concept that usually implies deliberate wrongdoing. It is worth stating emphatically that in this situation no one is at fault, not the child or teenager, not parents, not teachers. Once parents and teachers have a more complete understanding of the causes of a child's lack of school success, they often feel deep regret and remorse for the angry, accusatory things they have said in the past.

Step Two: You stop what you are doing and listen attentively.

The child may be complaining, whingeing, arguing or even crying. Sometimes he is silent but his facial expression and body language speak volumes: a scowl of fury, a dejected slouch, brows knitted in worry. You can show you are listening by responding with: 'Oh . . . mmm . . . I see.' This helps the child start to relax and feel safe, whereas asking 'What's the matter?' often puts an inarticulate child on the spot and results in a shrug and 'I don't know,' or possibly a torrent of blame.

Step Three: You imagine what your child is feeling below the level of his words, and you reflect back to the child in words what you imagine he is feeling, rather than trying to argue him out of his version of reality.

'This is stupid' often means, *'This worksheet looks too hard.'*

'Go away,' or *'Don't look at me,'* or *'Leave me alone,'* might mean, *'I'm afraid I'll lose my temper if you keep talking to me,'* or possibly, *'I'm ashamed that I keep making mistakes.'*

'I hate maths' could really mean, *'I don't understand what the teacher says, and she gets annoyed with me if I ask.'*

You can say:

I can see you're upset. It's hard to settle down to homework when you'd rather be playing.

Maybe you're feeling that this maths is just too difficult and that you'll never understand it.

Even just thinking about revision seems to be getting you down.

Step Four is optional: You give your child his wishes in fantasy.

This often lightens the mood, and again it shows the child that you care and understand:

You probably wish you would never ever, ever have another spelling test again in your whole life.
What if you had a magical essay-writing pen that did all the work for you!

I wish I could make time fly so that you would be finished with your homework in three seconds.

To sum up, when a child is experiencing uncomfortable emotions, he often acts this out through subtle or not-so-subtle misbehaviour: arguing, complaining, time-wasting, refusing, breaking his pencil, storming off, etc. Knowing this, whenever the child is uncooperative we can choose to respond initially with Reflective Listening rather than by nagging, arguing back or shouting, which are all quite counterproductive and emotionally draining for the parent as well as the child.

Rewards

We cannot expect our children to simply accept our new routines and rules. Changing habits is difficult enough for adults. This is true even when we are absolutely convinced that a new habit would be good for us (for example, eating healthily or exercising). Children and teens, however, will not be at all convinced that the new homework habits will benefit them. And in addition, they are naturally reluctant to concentrate more carefully on an area of their lives where they do not currently feel comfortable or successful.

One way to motivate children is with little rewards that are easy and quick to deliver and cost nothing. You will be willing to give many of these little rewards every day, not just for excellent behaviour and homework habits (which you will not see every day), but also for small steps in the right direction, even when the results are still not quite what you were hoping for. The very easiest, quickest and most effective rewards are our positive reactions to every little improvement:

- Smiles
- Hugs
- Descriptive Praise
- Thumbs-up sign or other gesture of approval

These tiny rewards are very motivating, even for highly resistant children and teens.

In order to guide your children to develop the habit of doing their best, notice every time they make a better-than-average effort, and reward them immediately with those four easy, quick rewards, for example when they:

- Show you what their homework is the first time you ask
- Don't argue when you point out a mistake during the improving stage of homework
- Don't ask for screen time before their homework is completed to your satisfaction
- Sit at their homework for a few minutes longer than usual before popping up to pet the dog
- Explain to you the worked example in the text book, instead of ignoring it
- Don't say 'This is boring'

Remember that, deep down, children and teens want to please parents who are friendly and appreciative. So once you commit yourself to rewarding all the tiny steps in the right direction with Descriptive Praise and smiles, your children will soon be more and more motivated to do the right thing.

Extrinsic rewards are also very powerful. When we are expecting children to concentrate on something that does not particularly interest them or that they may feel is too difficult, it helps to offer a reward. The reward does not take the place of the Descriptive Praise, the *think-throughs* or the rules and routines. Rewards add an extra bit of motivation that helps children over the initial hump of their resistance. Rewards make it easier for children to get into good habits. You will find that you won't need to keep rewarding the same behaviour once it becomes a solid habit.

When thinking about homework, the purpose of the reward is to motivate children to concentrate better, write more neatly, answer questions more thoroughly, write something for each question rather than leaving blanks, not give up, etc. We are looking for progress, not perfection. Your child should be able to earn the rewards on offer by demonstrating more willingness than before or by producing work that's a bit better than her previous work.

Children, particularly the more sensitive, intense, impulsive ones, are often asking us for something, either directly or indirectly:

Will you fix this for me?

Can I have another biscuit?

Will you play with me?

If you want to respond to a particular request with 'Yes,' it is helpful to turn your reply into an instant reward that reinforces the homework habits you value. You could say:

Yes, I'd be glad to help you because you really slowed down and were so careful with your handwriting today. You kept most of your letters on the line.

Yes, I'll be happy to take the time to sit down and fix this for you. I want to because I'm so pleased with how you've been cooperating about homework. You thought you couldn't do tens-and-units, but you tried and you tried and you didn't give up. And you got most of them right.

Using screen time as a reward

Most children spend some time every day in front of a screen, whether it's a television, computer, Wii, Xbox, iPad or mobile phone. Because screens are so mesmerising and most children and teens love them, I recommend that children have to earn their daily screen time by completing their homework to the parents' satisfaction, by doing some household chores and by being friendly and cooperative. If your child is currently quite dependent on screens he may be very upset to learn that he is going to have to earn something he assumed was his birthright. Prepare for Success by telling him a week or so in advance what the new rule will be, and do several *think-throughs* a day, asking him to tell you all about the new rule. You can ask him what he needs to do to earn his screen time, where he has to do his homework, how much screen time he can earn and why you have made this new rule. If you are willing to do several *think-throughs* a day, you will soon see his resistance starting to melt.

If your child or teen is really hooked on electronics, at first you may need to Prepare for Success by making sure you have all the remotes and the chargers in your possession. You may even need to remove a wire from the back of the computer, and you will almost certainly need to put a password on the computer and to block certain websites during the homework time.

Whenever I suggest this radical step of having screen time be earned, parents have many questions and concerns. Parents often feel helpless and powerless; they assume that they cannot get back in charge of their children's screen use. You can! In my earlier book, *Calmer, Easier, Happier Parenting*, I address these worries.

Some families don't have daily screen time, so this reward would not be relevant. But there are always things children want to do or have. Make it clear that children can earn these activities, such as using coloured markers, using arts and crafts materials, playing with a special train set, or playing a board game with a parent.

Once your child has earned her reward for the day, do not threaten to take it away from her, even if she misbehaves later. She has earned the reward, and it is hers. If you feel the need to give consequences for other misbehaviour, deal with that infraction separately.

Rewards help children and teens get used to new rules. Once these are established as habits, the rewards will no longer be necessary. In *Calmer, Easier Happier Parenting*, the companion volume to this book, I explain in more detail how parents can use different types of rewards to foster good habits.

Consequences

At any given moment during the daily homework session, a child is either cooperating with the routines and rules, or he is not cooperating. I know that it can be tempting to ignore little bits of misbehaviour, a bit of rule bending or a slightly disrespectful tone of voice. There are lots of reasons parents give me for choosing to look the other way:

- You worry that correcting your child may trigger more misbehaviour, which would delay getting the homework done and cause even more problems.
- The minor misbehaviour doesn't really seem that important, as long as the child is still working.
- You're following the often-quoted advice, 'Pick your battles'. The misbehaviour seems minor, and you want to save your energy for dealing with major misbehaviour.

However, if we want our children to respect us and to take our routines and rules seriously, we need to respond consistently and immediately to <u>all</u> instances of non-cooperation. This means not only the major, but also the minor infractions. Not only the deliberate misbehaviour, but also the impulsive, compulsive and habitual. Not only the breaking of rules, but also the bending of rules.

Why parents are often reluctant to follow through with consequences

When parents have not yet discovered the almost magical power of consistency, they tend to apply sanctions in a rather haphazard manner, based on their mood, how tired they are that day or how upset they already are about something else. Sadly, parents do not realise that inconsistent responses often perpetuate misbehaviour. The parents end up assuming that consequences don't work for their child.

Parents are often reluctant to *follow through* consistently after misbehaviour because they believe that consequences will result in even more whingeing, sulking, tears, tantrums, refusals and verbal aggression. That is occasionally true in the first week or so of your new, more consistent approach. Sometimes things do get worse before they get better. So persevere!

Another reason parents are often hesitant to consistently *follow through* is because they worry that they would come across as harsh, tyrannical or uncaring. When we choose, for these reasons or for any other, to ignore subtle or minor misbehaviour, the child gradually loses respect for what we say, which results, over time, in more and more uncooperative behaviour. Parents try to be patient, but, being human, eventually they snap, reacting with blame, threats and shouting. Ironically, parental reluctance to immediately address each incident results in parents speaking and acting in more negative, unfriendly ways that children do often perceive as harsh, tyrannical or uncaring. Erratic consequences or sudden outbursts are likely to breed resentment and anxiety, whilst consistent consequences soon lead to a more relaxed, more confident, motivated, better-behaved child or teenager.

Consequences are most effective when they are mild rather than severe, when they are over with quickly and when they happen every time a rule is broken. The first rule for parents is: Take immediate action. Action means doing, not saying. So do not repeat yourself or remind, cajole, threaten, argue or bargain. All of those responses will only prolong the problem.

Three consequences that parents have used successfully to help transform homework habits

Remove the homework

Paradoxically, when a child is sitting in front of his homework, but not working properly or not working at all, whether he is complaining or staring into space for long minutes at a time, a useful consequence is to remove his books, paper, pencil case and any other equipment.

You might think your child would be delighted with this turn of events, interpreting your action as letting him off the hook. Interestingly, the opposite is true. When the space in front of him on the homework table is suddenly empty, he cannot continue to fool himself that he is doing his homework. It soon hits home that there is no longer a grey area where he can pretend to himself that he is working.

It is important for parents not to threaten this. Instead, Prepare for Success earlier in the day by having several *think-throughs*, during which you explain the new plan in a couple of sentences (no lecturing, please!) and then ask your child to tell you exactly what will happen if you judge that he is not working properly. Then, if the time-wasting happens again, take immediate action, as soon as necessary.

Do not be tempted to give him back his books as soon as he promises to follow your instructions or to do his work carefully. Instead, wait until you can <u>see</u> and <u>hear</u>, from his tone of voice, his facial expression and even his posture, that he is completely ready to do his best. At that point, do yet another *think-through*. Have him tell you exactly what he will do and how he will do it. Getting to this point may take longer than you wish it would! But this is how we establish more sensible habits.

Very occasionally, a stubborn child will waste so much

time before she is ready to cooperate and do her homework properly that it cannot be completed within the allotted time. Do not let her work any later than the time allotted for it, as I explained in Chapter 5. If you like, you can send a note in to the teacher briefly explaining what you did, and then let your child take whatever consequence the school gives her. Above all, stay positive. Children learn quickly from consequences when we stay calm and don't blame. But as soon as we get angry or even annoyed, the child gets angry right back and is no longer motivated to do what he knows he should do.

Do an action replay

An *action replay* is a particularly useful consequence, whether the misbehaviour was impulsive, compulsive, habitual or deliberate.

In an *action replay*, you and your child replay the scene, but this time he says or does the right thing. For example, if he called you an insulting name, this time he says how he feels, just as strongly, but using polite words. If he threw his pencil across the room, in the *action replay* he will handle his frustration more maturely, perhaps by making a request for a short break or by taking several deep breaths. If he refused to do his homework, saying, 'I'm stupid,' in the *action replay* he will have another go at the sum that seemed too difficult, and this time take a sensible guess.

Before you ask your child to do the *action replay*, wait for him to calm down. This usually takes only a few minutes, but it might even take a few hours at first, especially if your child has a trickier, more intense temperament or if he has been feeling angry or discouraged about homework for a long time.

No reward for the day

If we shift our focus from indulging to rewarding, a very effec-tive consequence is that the child has not earned his reward that day.

For example, the rule might be that he can earn an hour of screen time every evening by completing his homework within the allotted time (if the homework your child is set is too diffi-cult for him to complete within the allotted time, see Chapter 7 for what you can do). If he wastes time and therefore does not complete the homework to your satisfaction, he has not earned that evening's screen time. For the child, this is not the same as the withdrawal of an entitlement to screen time. With this new approach he cannot take it for granted that he will be able to go on the computer every evening; he knows that he must earn it daily.

The tools that I have described in this chapter are not magic wands. But over time, and sooner than you would imagine, these Calmer, Easier, Happier Parenting strategies will help improve your child's cooperation, confidence, motivation, self-reliance and consideration.

CHAPTER 7

TYPICAL HOMEWORK PROBLEMS AND SOLUTIONS

A few years ago, when my middle child was about seven, her teacher was complaining that she wasn't concentrating in class. And at home we were noticing that she'd got into the habit of saying 'No' to just about everything, not just homework. She has one of those intense temperaments anyway, but she seemed to be getting worse. I'd heard somewhere about Calmer, Easier, Happier Parenting so I googled it to see if they could help with Sarah's concentration problem. The advice I got was so practical and straightforward. We realised that the maths was too difficult for her because she hadn't memorised her addition and subtraction bonds. So we did the micro-skills; we practised the bonds for five minutes a day. In just a week or two the teachers said she was already much better. And she was paying attention and putting her hand up. We were so happy. We also realised that she used to say 'I don't know,' a lot, and her older sisters would explain everything to her. So we sat down with the older children and asked them not to do that any more so that Sarah could learn to think for herself. We did lots of think-throughs and of course we did Descriptive Praise for every tiny little thing; she just lapped it up. It's hard to remember how worried we were about her. She's twelve now and she's so motivated and proud of herself when she does well.

Mother of four, two older teens,
a 12-year-old girl and a 7-year-old boy

All children sometimes complain about homework and sometimes look for excuses to put it off until later. The real problems arise when children <u>habitually</u> resist doing their best or resist doing homework altogether. Parents want to understand why their child regularly makes a fuss about doing homework or takes a long time to settle down, and they want to know what they can do to foster willingness and improve concentration. It is worth taking the time to see which of the following problems apply, as that will help us identify the solutions.

1 **Problem** Your child may be motivated to do his homework, but regularly finds that the work is genuinely too difficult for him. He resists in an understandable attempt to avoid frustration, embarrassment and feeling like a failure.

   Solution Here is what to do when you can clearly see that a piece of homework is too difficult for your child:

   • Reflectively Listen to your child about how this situation might make him feel (see Chapter 6).

   • Do not do his thinking for him; do not do any part of the work for him. That would mask the problem.

   • Do not simply require him to do less of it. That would not address the real problem, which is that he needs to master certain skills.

   • Make a unilateral decision to simplify the homework so that he can be and feel successful, but do <u>not</u> let him just leave it undone. For a child with good listening comprehension whose reading skills are still weak, you can often make the homework do-able by reading aloud to him the instructions, worksheet or textbook passage. As you read each sentence aloud, slowly, with exaggerated expression, require your child first to follow along with his finger, and then to re-read each sentence aloud correctly by himself as you slowly point to each word. He will be able to achieve this quite easily because the words he has just heard you read will still be very fresh in his mind. At first, he may be parroting most of the sentence, rather than actually decoding, but this technique serves several very useful purposes:

- Seeing and hearing the words simultaneously will soon improve your child's reading skills.
- He will experience himself as a reader, which will enhance his confidence and motivation.
- He will stay actively involved in his homework, rather than sitting back and expecting you to explain it to him.

• Give him lots of practice at an easier level and Descriptively Praise even tiny improvements.

• Do not let your child leave any answers blank. He needs to take a guess and write something, even if he is not sure whether his answer is right. Only then can the teacher assess where he is going wrong.

• Do not keep urging your child to ask the teacher for help. Many children with school problems are too embarrassed to ask. Or else they know from past experience that the teacher's explanation will not clarify matters sufficiently.

• Make sure that the teachers know when your child is experiencing problems and how you are tackling them. For example, if you are reading the homework instructions aloud to your child, you need to make sure his teachers know this. Otherwise they will continue to expect more of him than he is currently capable of producing.

• Be a staunch advocate for your child. Learn everything you can about the possible causes of his academic or behaviour problems and about useful strategies for home and school. Then share what you have learned with his teachers (without, of course, directly telling them what to do).

2 **Problem** Your child regularly forgets to bring home his homework.

Solution A child who regularly forgets to bring home his homework diary, worksheets and books will of course find his homework confusing and difficult. This child can learn to remember, although at first he may not believe he can. Teachers can help a dreamy or impulsive pupil to get into the habit of remembering to take home what he needs. At home, *think-throughs* and rewards are often very effective for these children.

We should not be surprised or shocked that some children have developed the habit of deliberately leaving their homework at school or conveniently misplacing it. These are children who experience homework as an ordeal to be avoided at all costs. When parents start to establish enjoyable, productive homework routines, it becomes easier and easier for these children to do the right thing.

KEY CONCEPT

When the homework itself is the problem

Unfortunately, a lot of the homework that children and teens are set is not fit for purpose. Homework should reinforce skills and information that children already understand. Children should not be given homework that requires them to use skills or information that they have not thoroughly learned at school, but too often that is what happens. And too often homework makes no attempt to capture the interest of the student. This can unintentionally reinforce unproductive habits because the child is tempted to rush through it to get it over with.

In addition, the way returned homework is dealt with is often unproductive. The teacher frequently puts in quite a lot of effort with a red pen, marking the mistakes. The assumption must be that pupils will study these red marks and learn from them how to do things better the next time. But it is the rare child (or even adult) who is motivated to study a teacher's comments on what he did wrong. So the teacher's efforts are largely wasted. Some teachers require pupils to rewrite the homework, taking into account the teacher's comments. This is where true learning can take place, but unfortunately this rarely happens.

3 **Problem** Your child often doesn't know what the homework is.

Solution It can be tempting to blame the teacher for this, assuming that he or she has not explained the homework properly. This assumption will not hold water if other pupils in the class <u>do</u> understand how to do the homework.

The problem here may be that your child has real difficulty writing the homework down accurately or fast enough so she is confused when the time comes to do her homework. This is not the child's fault. Parents will need to be advocates for their child to ensure that the teacher takes appropriate action. The teacher might:

- Write the homework instructions in the child's homework diary for her.
- Give the child written homework instructions for her to copy into her homework diary. This will probably be much easier for her than copying from the board, which requires a continual big shift in visual focus as the board is much farther away.
- At the very least, write the homework instructions on

the board much earlier in the lesson, so that the child has more time to copy neatly and accurately rather than having to rush to get it all copied in the last few minutes before the bell rings.

4 **Problem** Your child seems quite capable of doing a good job on his homework, but only after you have explained the instructions or briefly retaught some of the concepts.

Solution If a child <u>often</u> seems to need to have instructions clarified or concepts retaught, parents tend to jump to incorrect conclusions. You may blame your child for not having bothered to listen carefully during the lesson. However, she may have written down the teacher's oral instructions incorrectly because she cannot easily listen, understand and write all at the same time. Below are some likely reasons why a child might not be listening carefully to the teacher:

- The child may be easily distracted by background noise. This pupil is, in fact, listening as carefully as his brain currently knows how to listen, given the many auditory and visual distractions of a noisy, busy classroom. The child with this problem may complain that his classmates are too noisy and may even blame the teacher for not knowing how to keep the class quiet.

- The child may be relatively immature or impulsive and therefore find it difficult to sustain attention on a topic that does not particularly interest him.

- He may be a kinaesthetic learner who pays attention best when he is actively involved, but finds it hard to sustain attention when he must sit still and passively take in information.

- He may not be able to process the information as quickly as the teacher is talking, which is one of the signs of an auditory processing problem. Once he loses the thread, the teacher's words become confusing or meaningless, and can seem boring.

- He may not know how to focus on the important details of what the teacher is saying. This child may be able to regale you with statistics or examples, while missing the main points of the lesson. He, too, may become confused and bored; soon his mind wanders.

- Your child may have a relatively poor short-term auditory memory; he very quickly forgets what he hears.

- He may not understand the subject terminology, which once again results in confusion and boredom, as well as a belief that the subject or topic is too hard.

- He may not have really mastered the previous lessons on this topic, so he does not have the foundation with which to make sense of the new information. Without even realising it, he switches off.

In Chapter 14, I explain how parents can improve a child's listening comprehension. This can go a long way towards ironing out the above problems.

5 **Problem** Your child frequently asks for help with her homework.

Solution Sometimes when a child asks for help she wants an explanation of how to do something, but sometimes she actually wants the parent to tell her the answer. She is hoping that the parent's brain will do the work, probably because the parent has done too much for her in the past. We must not fall into the trap of doing our children's thinking for them. So whenever you feel the urge to explain, do the following instead:

- Ask leading questions rather than telling your child. Only when <u>her</u> brain has to come up with the answer is she learning.

- Draw pictures and diagrams, using a minimum of words, because, as we have seen, many children with school problems are strong visual learners and weak auditory learners.
- Give lots of examples so that your child can see for herself what they all have in common.
- Reflectively Listen to her frustration and confusion.
- Descriptively Praise her whenever she thinks for herself.

Specifically for mathematics:

- Talk your child through a sum that is similar to the one he has to do for his homework. That way, once he understands the principle or procedure from your explanation, he will still have to use his own brain to work out the sum he was given for homework.
- Give examples that use much, much easier numbers so that the child can concentrate solely on the procedures or principles.

6 **Problem** Your child may be avoiding a particular type of homework because he thinks he can't do it or thinks he can't do it well enough, even though you are sure he could do it if he would just stop complaining and start concentrating. This child is often a perfectionist with a sensitive temperament. He would rather be told off for making a fuss than risk disappointing his parents or teachers by getting it wrong.

OR

7 **Problem** Your child may be able to do his homework, but is just trying to get out of doing it. He knows from past experience that if he makes enough of a fuss his parents will sometimes give in, and he will end up working less and playing more.

Solution For both of these causes of resistance, the strategies to use are the same:

- Reflectively Listen about his anxieties or his lack of confidence or his resentments.
- Prepare for Success by doing *think-throughs*, several times a day, about the new plan to divide the homework into three stages (see Chapter 5). He needs to be able to tell you that in Stage One you will ask questions to help him remember everything he needs to know and that in Stage Two he will need to do all of his homework on his own. Make sure he knows that you will not get angry if he makes mistakes. You can do a one-minute *think-through* over breakfast, another *think-through* on the way to school and another on the way home from school.
- Remember, you know he <u>can</u> do it. Do not simplify the homework or do part of it for him 'to get him started' or even read the instructions to him. That would send him the message that you do not think him capable.
- Do not allow him to do less.
- Stay positive and friendly as you insist that he does it.
- Give lots of Descriptive Praise, especially for willingness, courage and determination.

8 **Problem** Your child may understand the work and be capable of giving very reasonable verbal responses, but he is trying to avoid writing, which he finds difficult to do well, very time-consuming or even physically painful.
  Solution If this is happening:
- Recognise that some children find writing physically, and therefore emotionally, uncomfortable.
- Reflectively Listen to how he feels about writing, about schoolwork, homework, his teachers, his abilities, etc.
- He and you may need several sessions with an

occupational therapist or handwriting specialist, who will show you exercises for him to do at home every day to:
- Strengthen his muscles
- Improve his posture, the position of his arms and the way he holds his pencil
- Form his letters correctly

An occupational therapist will also tell you if your child would benefit from specially adapted equipment, such as a wedge-shaped board to place his work on or a moulded pencil grip that guides his fingers into a more comfortable and more effective position.

In Chapter 19, I talk more about what parents can do to improve handwriting.

KEY CONCEPT

Why do more boys struggle with homework than girls?

Certain skills tend to mature more slowly in boys than in girls. At least into adolescence, boys are likely to be more active, restless and have problems with impulse-control, whereas girls of the same age are more able to sit still and listen quietly for longer periods.

Girls' language also develops earlier, with the result that they tend to speak in longer and more complex sentences that have extra clauses. They use more adjectives, which makes their language easier to understand. Their vocabulary tends to be richer too, in the sense that they regularly use different words within a category to make distinctions.

Fine motor skills are another area where boys tend to lag behind girls. In terms of schoolwork and homework, this affects handwriting, drawing, using a ruler, making diagrams, etc.

Boys tend to have lots of physical energy, with the result that they want to move around a lot, and this gets them told off in the classroom. Boys tend to be more daring and to enjoy physical risk-taking; this also gets them into trouble in the classroom.

However, not all differences between boys and girls are purely the result of nature. We know that from birth boys and girls are treated differently in every culture. It has been shown that in our culture girls are spoken to more and parents make more eye contact with girls, whereas parents are more likely to draw a boy infant's attention to an object. Certainly boys and girls tend to be given different toys and are expected to be interested in different activities, although that is slowly changing.

Most boys are raised by women, who are often impatient with the noisy, active ways of boys. Because most teachers, especially in primary school, are women, classrooms are better suited to girls' development. As a result, boys can start to feel, from an early age, that they are annoying or 'bad', even that there is something wrong with them. In fact, the American psychologist Michael Thompson has written that in schools boys are treated as defective girls. Too often this results in boys developing quite a negative attitude towards school in general and towards teachers in particular. None of this bodes well for homework going smoothly!

9 **Problem** Your child knows how to do his homework, but is not in the habit of doing his best.

Solution If your child understands his homework and knows how to do it, but regularly rushes or dawdles through his work, not doing his best, he will need to improve his attention to detail in one, or possibly all, of the following areas:

- Accuracy
- Thoroughness
- Presentation

Expect your child to argue and complain:

This is science, so spelling doesn't matter.

The teacher doesn't care if it's neat as long as the answer is right.

I don't have time to write that much.

You think I have to be perfect.

You're not my teacher.

Sometimes complaints are phrased as questions, the favourites being: 'Why do I have to?' and 'What does it matter?' These are not really questions that your child wants answers to! Remember that you are in charge. Your standard, not the child's and not even the school's, is what your child needs to be striving to reach. So don't argue back. Instead:

- Reflectively Listen to how he might be feeling.
- Thorough Stage One *think-throughs* (see Chapter 5) every day will very quickly start to improve the quality of his work by focusing his attention on the standard you require.
- Make a rule that every piece of weekend homework must be done in rough first. (Your child will probably not have enough time on school nights to do this consistently.) That way the final copy will be a piece of work that your child can be proud of.
- Descriptively Praise all improvements in willingness as well as work.

10 **Problem** Your child may have picked up from you some subtle clues that you secretly believe the teacher is not worthy of respect. **Solution** To help your child respect the teachers' and the school's rules and policies:

- Never let your child overhear you saying anything even remotely critical about the teachers, homework, school policies, etc. If you do, you will unintentionally be giving him tacit permission not to take school seriously.
- Instead, write down your criticisms or complaints as requests, and then address them to the person who could, in theory, do something about your request.
- Descriptively Praise everything you can about the school.

KEY CONCEPT

The language that parents use

The language that we use is never neutral. We are always sending out some kind of message with the words we speak, either intentionally or unintentionally. It makes sense for us to put some thought into intentionally sending positive messages. We want to use language that shows that we know our children are capable of learning and that homework does not have to be an ordeal.

The first word I want to look at is the word '**help**'. This is a tricky word because it means different things at different times. Unfortunately some of the ways we use the word 'help' can be very disempowering:

- One of the dictionary definitions of the word 'help' is to make it easier for someone to do something. As parents, the only reason we would want to make homework easier is if it is too difficult. But as long as it is not too difficult, the child should be doing it by herself with no help from us.

- Another dictionary definition of 'help' is to improve a situation or problem, to make it better or less painful. There are definitely ways that we can improve homework and make it less painful and more enjoyable. That is what this book is about.

- Another definition of the word 'help' is to do part of another person's work for him. Homework is intended to be done by the child. But most of the time when we talk about 'helping' children with their homework, we mean doing for them some part of the work that they should be doing for themselves. This sends a disempowering message.

- Yet another meaning of the word 'help' is to do something with or for someone that he cannot do alone. That makes sense as long as at the same time we are teaching the child how to do it for himself, so that in time he will not need the help.

- And 'help' also means to do something with or for someone that he will find useful. It is _not_ useful for us to do something for our child that he can do for himself.

You can see from all these definitions that the meanings overlap and range from a useful action that will benefit someone all the way to actions that would not be good. To avoid confusion, I recommend that as much as possible we replace the word 'help' with words that are more specific and more accurate.

When a child asks 'Can you help me?' we need to think about what the child needs, not what he wants. Maybe we need to be teaching a micro-skill or training a habit. Possibly we will simply be sitting with the child to keep him company if he can do the work by himself but thinks he cannot due to anxiety or a lack of self-confidence. We might be demonstrating how to do something. We might be asking questions. It is the premise of this book that the best way we can 'help' with homework is to learn and put into practice the core strategies that I talk about in Chapter 5 and the specific strategies I talk about in the other chapters.

Another phrase that we need to be careful about is '**working hard**'. Parents will often say, 'You've been working so hard,' or, 'You really need to work harder'. There are two problems with this phrase. The first is that children tend to be very literal, so when they hear the word 'hard' they automatically think 'difficult'. Without realising it, parents are unintentionally reinforcing the idea that homework is difficult. The other problem with the phrase 'working hard' is that it is far too vague to be useful to the child. Let's be more specific. You could Descriptively Praise:

You didn't feel like sitting down and doing this, but you stopped complaining and you're halfway through already.

When you weren't sure what the answers were, you didn't leave any blanks. You took a sensible guess, and you wrote something down.

You spent two hours revising your French vocab over the weekend. That took determination!

From Descriptive Praises like these your child can see what actions you value, and you will find that he is motivated to do more and more of what you are noticing and mentioning. This is how he learns to 'work hard'.

Another word to avoid is '**lazy**'. It is easy to use the word 'lazy' as shorthand for a child who is not making her best effort. The problem with the word 'lazy' is that it suggests that there is no good reason for the child's behaviour or attitude. The word 'lazy' implies that she is not bothering simply because she doesn't feel like it. In my experience this is very far from the truth. When children are just going through the motions and not doing their best, or when they are trying to avoid doing their work altogether, there is always a reason. We need to discover and address the reason. That is what this book is all about.

You are likely to hear the word '**boring**' quite a lot at homework time until more enjoyable and productive habits are established. Nowadays many children expect to be entertained. The word 'boring' in relation to homework can mean that it looks too hard. Often 'boring' means that it is not entertaining, not particularly interesting, not what children would choose to do if they had a choice, and therefore they don't want to do it. Those are all legitimate feelings, but using the word 'boring' is very misleading. When your child says maths is boring, the implication is that it is a fact that maths is boring. But it's simply not true. Some people find maths boring and some people find maths fascinating. That is true of every single school subject. Therefore, there is no such thing as 'boring' as a fact. So when children say something is 'boring', let's remember to Reflectively Listen to the feeling behind the words:

Maybe it feels like there are too many sums on this page.

It's a sunny day, and you'd rather be on your skateboard.

It's been a while since you did fractions, and maybe you're not sure you remember how to do them.

I am not suggesting that we correct or reprimand our children when they use the word 'boring'. What I am recommending is that we do not use the word ourselves, <u>ever</u>. Let's set a good example. And let's remember to Reflectively Listen to the real feelings below the surface.

11 **Problem** Your child may have an important concert or sports event that means she doesn't have time to complete all her homework.
   Solution There will be times when, for various reasons, all the homework won't get done. So go for quality over quantity. Focus on what *you* think are the most important tasks.

CHAPTER 8

COMPUTERS, TUTORS AND WORKBOOKS: HELP OR HINDRANCE?

> *I used to get upset when I saw my children doing their homework by downloading information from articles on the internet, just changing a few words and then printing it out. They said that was what all the kids did. They couldn't see that it was wrong. And half the time they didn't even really understand what they printed out. I decided to stop arguing and trying to convince them. My husband and I made some new rules. They could read whatever they needed from the various websites and they could make brief notes, but then they had to go into the dining room, where there was no computer, and write their homework from their notes and from whatever they remembered they had read. It took a few weeks for them to get over thinking that we were the stupidest parents in the whole world. We did lots of Descriptive Praise and Reflective Listening and Preparing for Success. That was almost a year ago, and they still do their homework that way. I'm so relieved because now I know that they're really thinking and learning, not just copying.*
>
> Mother of two, aged 13 and 11

The use of computers

Older children will often want, and may actually need, to use the computer for homework and projects. Unsupervised, this can easily degenerate into surreptitious playing of computer games, chatting online, emailing their friends, checking Facebook or surfing the net, then quickly switching the screen back to their homework as soon as you enter the room. One way to prevent this from happening is to keep all screens in areas of the house that you can easily supervise and to take immediate action if you even suspect misuse. In addition, if misuse is a problem, use all the mechanical and electronic methods now available to put various computer functions off limits during the *sacred homework time*.

You may also need a rule with a consequence. Make and stick to a rule that any misuse of the computer automatically means that the child has not earned the right to use the computer, for homework or for pleasure, for the next few days. You may feel sorry for him and want to relent when he complains that your *following through* with a consequence will result in a detention or the teacher marking his work down. But remember that he is the one who broke the rule; he brought the consequence on himself. Equally, don't get angry when he breaks the rule. Some amount of rule breaking is a natural part of growing up. Our responses to rule breaking will determine whether the rule breaking gradually escalates or whether it gradually fades away. Instead of lecturing, 'It's your own fault', we can show that we care about the child's feelings: 'It sounds like you're worried that you'll get into trouble. You're probably wishing you hadn't broken the computer rule'.

A typical problem is that your child or teenager may print out pages and pages of information from the internet and hand it in as his own work. At the higher levels of academic study, plagiarism is a crime. Even when that is not a concern, passing off someone else's work as his own allows the child to avoid using his brain, and it allows him to not take the homework seriously. It is, therefore, the parents' job to insist that children put everything into their own words. Expect resistance at first!

If this has become a problem, you can use the three stages of homework to teach and train better habits:

Stage One: The *think-through*

- Decide for yourself whether the computer is necessary for this piece of homework. Do not take your child's word for it.
- By asking questions, not by telling, guide your child to understand why he should not take credit for what another person has produced.
- He also needs to understand that one of the teacher's purposes, in setting the class a particular essay or project, is to give pupils practice in learning to think for themselves. Printing out someone else's work is the opposite of thinking for himself.
- To teach him what to do instead of handing in someone else's work as his own, require your child or teenager to think about and jot down an outline of what he will write. Once he realises that he has a fair idea of the key points he needs to cover, he will be more confident and therefore less tempted to pad his essay or project with reams of someone else's work.
- Make sure he knows that in Stage Three you will be checking to see that he has put everything from the text-book or from the internet into his own words, not just changed a phrase here and there.

Stage Two: Your child works on her own

Your child should now work on his homework without any help.

Stage Three: The improving stage

Check to see whether he has written about the key points that he jotted down during the *think-through* and whether he has used his own words.

Tutors

Last year my son managed to persuade us that he needed a tutor for French and for maths. He said his teachers were no good at controlling the class so nobody could get any work done. We believed him so we arranged for the tutors, which was expensive. We asked both the tutors to give Andy homework every week. At first he argued about the extra homework, but he soon saw that he could do the maths homework quite easily because the tutor had explained it step by step so Andy understood what he had to do. After about a month, Andy was feeling confident about the maths. And suddenly there were no more complaints about the teacher! So we stopped the maths tutor, and Andy was fine. The French tutor was not so successful. Even after a month of tutoring, Andy was just as confused and negative about French as ever. I think that tutor wasn't so good at explaining things, and he didn't smile much, which didn't help. There was no rapport. So we stopped the French tutor as well after a month, but for the opposite reason. Then my wife and I took turns sitting with Andy whenever he was doing his French homework, quizzing him, getting him to explain the conjugations to us. And we always made him do his French homework first, before he got too tired. It was fun, actually. And he got much better. Even though I can't speak French and neither can my wife, working with him is what made all the difference. So we've had a mixed experience when it comes to tutors.

Father of boy, aged 14

It is becoming more and more common for parents to turn to tutors when children are having problems at school or with homework. Sometimes this turns out to be a satisfactory solution, especially if the tutor is willing to go back to basics, to reteach subjects starting at the child's current skill levels, rather than starting at the level the rest of the class has achieved. But often parents end up paying a lot of money without seeing lasting benefits.

Hiring a tutor can mask problems, particularly if the tutor is helping the child with homework. The homework that is turned in to the school cannot really be said to be the child's work because he could not have done it on his own.

Tutors, like teachers, are usually experts in their subject and usually they were good students themselves. Consequently, they often do not understand why a child is getting stuck or how to simplify a topic or skill to help the child get unstuck. Often they do not know how to motivate a child to be brave enough to concentrate on something that feels uncomfortable.

In a tutoring session, when a child says she does not understand something, the tutor is likely to simply re-explain. And because tutoring is usually one-to-one, tutors are able to keep re-explaining the same concepts week after week. When this happens the child is not learning how to marshal the information she does have and take a sensible guess. Without *attempting to retrieve* (which I talk about in Chapter 11), not much will be transferred into the long-term memory.

Anther problem is that tutors are employed by parents and naturally want to satisfy their employers. Therefore, they may tell the parent, and they may actually believe, that the child is improving more than he really is. Also, if the tutoring is weekly or even twice-weekly, there are still a number of days in between tutoring sessions in which the child can easily forget what he has been taught, unless parents review the information with the child daily. And if parents are willing to review daily, it is unlikely that a tutor will be needed.

Sometimes, with the help of a tutor, a child manages to hang in at a school that is actually too academic for him to be able to cope on his own. In that situation, the child will continue to need the tutor for as long as he is attending that school. This can undermine a child's confidence. And finally, tutors are expensive. Instead of assuming that a tutor is necessary, we need to get to the root of the problem so that we can decide what is needed. That is what this book is about.

Workbooks

We've used workbooks with our children, on and off, to supplement their schoolwork, especially during the long summer holidays. We didn't want their brains to shrivel up. And we used workbooks a lot when they were preparing for entrance exams. But two of my children, the boys, are quite slapdash and messy, always rushing to finish, and I was annoyed and frustrated. So my husband and I decided to follow Noël's advice. We taught them how to do their best, how to slow down and really pay attention to the instructions and how to do more than just the bare minimum. We gave them lots of little rewards, and Descriptive Praise of course, whenever they got a whole double page completely right, including neat handwriting. And that happened more and more because they loved the rewards. That was a few years ago. We still use workbooks with the younger two, but we don't need rewards any more because they're in the habit of doing their best now, not just in the workbooks but with all their homework and revision. Their marks improved steadily, and they're so proud of themselves.

Mother of three, aged 16, 12 and 10

When no homework has been set, whether during the term or the holidays, parents often turn to commercial workbooks. These can be an excellent way to reinforce skills, or they can be a waste of time and money. Here are my guidelines for how to use workbooks most effectively:

- Children tend to treat workbooks rather like toys, assuming they can use them how they like. As with term-time homework, you are in charge, and you decide the rules and routines for the homework habits you want your children to develop.
- When buying workbooks, choose a variety. Take your child with you when you go to buy them and allow her to have some input about which you will buy. But don't buy anything that you think is unsuitable. Make sure the workbooks are at the right level — not too easy or your child will not be stretched, but not too difficult or she will feel frustrated and won't learn much.
- For remedial work, choose workbooks intended for a younger child (as long as he is not insulted by too-childish graphics).
- Your child may assume that working in a workbook that you have bought for him is optional because the work was not set by the school. Remember that you're in charge. What you say goes.
- To reinforce their importance, call workbooks 'homework books', and keep them in a special place.
- If your child has several workbooks and prefers certain ones, make a rule that you decide which workbook she will work in every second day, and on the in between days, she can choose.
- Many workbook pages take very little time to do, so it's

a good idea to treat each double-page spread as one day's homework.

- Have your child start from the very beginning of each workbook and complete the whole of each double page (including writing the date and tackling any bonus questions) in the right order, rather than letting her choose whichever pages or exercises she thinks she will like the best or find the easiest.
- Draw 'handwriting lines' (a top line for tall letters and a halfway line for small letters) for any child whose handwriting is at all problematic. Workbooks rarely give children this important structure.
- Establish a rule that your child uses only pencil so that mistakes can be rubbed out and corrected.

Just as with school homework, divide each workbook task into the three stages:

Stage One: The *think-through*

- In addition to asking your child *think-through* questions about content and accuracy, also ask questions about neatness, thoroughness and presentation. Children often think these things don't matter in workbooks because the teacher won't be marking their work.
- Have your child estimate how long he thinks it will take him to do his best on the day's workbook task. Accurate estimating of time is a micro-skill that is essential for mature time management!
- Have your child use a highlighter to focus his attention on what he needs to think about on each page, eg noticing if sums are plus or minus or reading the instructions carefully.

Stage Two: Your child works on her own

Your child should now work in the workbook without any help.

Stage Three: The improving stage

Check to see that the work done in the workbook is of the same standard you would expect your child to produce for homework set by the school.

CHAPTER 9

IMPROVING YOUR CHILD'S LIFESTYLE CAN IMPROVE HOMEWORK HABITS

My daughter works long hours so my grandsons spend a lot of days and nights with me. Homework was a nightmare. And truthfully, so was the rest of the day, because they just didn't want to do what they were told. And they would egg each other on, getting sillier and wilder by the minute. The main thing I did differently from my daughter was to put them to bed a whole lot earlier on the nights they stayed over with me. That got rid of a lot of the grumpiness and the bickering between the two of them. I couldn't believe it. I also took advice from Noël's Homework DVD to give them a lot more exercise. I took them straight to the park after school and basically wore them out. Then when it was homework time, I didn't try and do homework with both of them together because that was just too difficult. I set it up so that while I was doing homework with one of the boys, the other one was playing independently the way Noël suggests. And then they switched. Suddenly, homework was fun for everybody. Before I learned these new strategies, I thought homework was a complete waste of time for four and five-year-olds. Now, I see how much they can learn in just fifteen minutes a day when they're really concentrating and not messing about.

Grandmother of two boys, aged 5 and 4

It's not just what happens during the daily homework time that influences how willing and able our children are to do their best academically. As parents, we create the largest part of our child's lifestyle. In this chapter, I would like to give some serious thought to how our family's lifestyle affects children, cognitively as well as physically and emotionally.

Bedtimes

When children and teenagers are regularly getting enough sleep, they do a better job on their homework. This is because a rested child is a better-behaved child. So even if your child's skill level is still lower than you would wish, once he is getting more sleep he is likely to be more willing and more cooperative.

Parents are often not aware of how much sleep children actually need in order to feel their best and do their best. Children and teens need more sleep than you realise, and they certainly need more sleep than <u>they</u> realise. Here are the guidelines I follow when advising parents about how many hours of sleep per night children need:

4-7 year olds: 11½ to 13 hours
7-10 year olds: 10½ to 12 hours
11-13 year olds: 9½ to 11 hours
13-14 year olds: 9½ to 10½ hours

In *Calmer, Easier, Happier Parenting* I explain how parents can establish and reinforce sensible bedtime habits. It is possible!

Nutrition

Many parents are aware that sugar makes their child overexcited, tearful, irritable or easily frustrated. What is not so widely known is that in sensitive children, sugar also adversely affects concentration, motivation, attention to detail, social awareness and short-term memory, all of which are essential school success skills.

Most parents know, in their hearts, that their children would be far better off with much less sugar. But parents worry that their children would complain bitterly if they had to do without and would feel that life was terribly unfair. Healthy eating need not be experienced, by children or by parents, as deprivation as long as you follow some important guidelines:

- Do not have the foods that are not good for them in the house so that the visual temptation is removed.
- Do not eat or drink any unhealthy foods in front of your children.
- Descriptively Praise them for their willingness, cooperation, flexibility, acceptance, etc.
- Reflectively Listen to how upset they may be feeling about the new healthy eating plan.
- Talk up the benefits of healthy food, but do not lecture them about unhealthy food.
- Allow a treat once or twice a week. Make sure that this happens outside the home to keep the boundaries clear.
- Allow them to eat what the other children are eating, without comment, at parties and on playdates.

Leisure activities (including screen time)

What children do during their free time, and even how much free time they have, has a big influence on the attitude with which they approach homework and revision.

When a child's day is tightly packed with after-school activities, even if those activities are very enjoyable, he ends up with very little time to just relax. This makes the idea of homework distinctly unappealing. As valuable as many after-school activities are, too many children are doing too much after school. Transfer some of those activities to weekends and holidays.

When children do have free time, they may spend a large part of that time in front of a screen, often before they settle down to their homework. Unfortunately, screen time saps motivation for homework. The less time children spend in front of a screen, the more cooperative and respectful and self-reliant they will become. I am not suggesting for a moment that all screens should be banned, although those few brave families who have taken the bold step of eliminating televisions, videos and computer games completely have not regretted it. Nowadays, that would not appeal to many parents.

But most parents I talk to are very keen to reduce the number of hours that their children and teens are spending in front of a screen. They also want to get back in charge of the quality and suitability of what their children are being exposed to.

Parents have reported many important benefits when children spend significantly less time in front of screens. Specifically in relation to homework:

- Children can concentrate for longer, and they develop the stamina to pursue activities that challenge them intellectually.
- Children are physically more active, which improves their posture, muscle tone, digestion and sleep habits. As a result, homework feels easier and less stressful.
- With less time spent in front of a screen, children talk more, which improves their vocabulary and sentence construction.

- Children put more energy and attention into all the other potentially enjoyable and rewarding activities that life has to offer: sport, practising a musical instrument, hobbies, playing with friends, cuddling or chatting with parents, quiet games, even homework and revision!
- They are more willing to read.
- They are more cooperative about doing their homework because they are less grumpy and irritable.
- When children have less exposure to on-screen aggression, intimidation, violence and destruction of property, their play gradually becomes less aggressive, less wild, even less competitive. This contributes to calmer homework.

To achieve these delightful results, we need to be determined and strong and brave. Getting back in charge of our children's screen time means bucking the trend of the past fifty years.

Based on the most up-to-date brain research, I advise that children up to the age of three years old have as little exposure to screens as possible. Between the ages of three and eight years old, it is recommended that children spend no more than half an hour a day in front of a screen. From the age of eight onwards, all the way through adulthood, the limit for leisure screen use should be an hour a day (except on special occasions, like going to the cinema or watching the World Cup).

This daily hour is for all screens combined, not an hour of videos and another hour on the computer and another hour playing on the DS! The daily hour of leisure screen time is separate from the time that children may need on the computer for homework. In Chapter 8, I explain about how parents can halt the misuse of the computer during homework time.

Exercise

When children can let off steam out-of-doors every day, they do less whingeing, crying and answering back. They concentrate better, they are less moody and more cheerful, and they have a higher tolerance for frustration. These are all qualities that are needed for school success and homework success, as well as for managing 'real life' more successfully. Some children, particularly boys and particularly those with a more difficult temperament, seem to have a much greater need than other children for lots of physical activity. This may feel too inconvenient to arrange, but it is an investment that pays off in calmer, more cooperative children and teens who will be able to focus, persevere and do their best, both at school and at homework time and in the rest of their lives.

Physical activity confers numerous benefits, all of which indirectly but significantly help a child to fulfil his academic potential:

- A child who gets plenty of exercise every day falls asleep more easily and sleeps more soundly, and therefore wakes more truly rested and refreshed. He is less irritable, less easily upset, more able to stay on task and to remember what is expected of him. This makes homework calmer, easier and happier.

- Vigorous physical activity also seems to help children who tend to be resistant or reluctant learners to 'burn off' some of their anger and their anxiety about schoolwork and homework.

- Fidgety, restless, impulsive children become significantly calmer and less 'hyper' when they have vigorous exercise every day. This calmness enables them to focus better and for longer.

The pace of a child's day

It is not fair to children to send them to a school that expects them to do homework and then not make a point of arranging their lives so that they can do their homework properly, when they are alert.

After-school activities often result in homework starting too late, when your child's brain is no longer fresh. She is less likely to be thinking clearly and more likely to make mistakes. As a result, homework can drag on and on, pushing bedtime back. The more tired children are, the more disorganised they are and the less self-confident they feel. So panic can set in, which makes falling asleep even harder.

One solution is to follow the rule I recommend in Chapter 5 about not letting homework take a minute longer than the school's guidelines. Another solution is to do as much homework in advance at the weekend as possible. You can expect your children to complain about this! Many families find that mornings are a good time to do homework, when children are rested and more alert. If these solutions do not work, it may be necessary to rearrange or cancel some of the after-school activities.

In *Calmer, Easier, Happier Parenting*, I explain in detail how you can use the five core strategies (Descriptive Praise, Preparing for Success, Reflective Listening, Never Ask Twice and Rewards and Consequences) to tackle the typical problems that parents often experience as they strive to maintain a healthy lifestyle for their family.

LEARNING HOW TO LEARN

CHAPTER 10

IMPROVING SELF-RELIANCE

> My two older children had both reacted to the birth of my third one by regressing. And even though the little one was already two years old, the older two were still acting helpless, especially about homework. Everything was 'I can't', 'I don't know how', 'It's too hard', 'You do it', 'Why do I have to?' Noël's recommendations on self-reliance were written just for me. We started by not answering their questions and making them take a guess. We Descriptively Praised whenever any of the children did things for themselves, even something as little as getting their own homework out of the homework bag. And we did lots of think-throughs. At first they wanted to answer all our questions with 'I don't know'. We Reflectively Listened, but we made them take a guess, and we Descriptively Praised them for being brave and taking a guess, even if the guesses weren't very good. And within a month they were so proud of themselves for using their own brains and for doing Stage Two of their homework from beginning to end without asking for help. And it wasn't just homework. They're now self-reliant about lots of other things too: getting dressed in the morning, putting their dishes in the sink, getting in and out of the bath by themselves. And they're more cooperative. These skills really work!
>
> Mother of three children, aged 8, 5 and 2

Infants start out very helpless so parents know that they have to do almost everything for them. Self-reliance naturally develops in stages as infants turn into toddlers and then into young children and then into older children and then into teenagers. But as children become able to do more and more for themselves, parents often get stuck at an earlier stage, doing things for children that they are now capable of doing for themselves. When it comes to homework, parents can even drift into the habit of doing their child's thinking for him.

Self-reliance is about a child taking responsibility for the things he is supposed to do. He is telling himself what he should do, rather than expecting someone else to do it for him, or rather than waiting until someone reminds him. A child or teen who is self-reliant is one who wants to do for himself everything that he can do for himself, and this includes taking pride in doing his best on his homework.

Self-reliance includes **organisation**, which is mostly about taking good care of one's belongings, keeping track of where they are and keeping them tidy. For example:

- Bringing home from school the right books, notes, worksheets, handouts, equipment, etc.
- Putting all completed homework in his book bag and putting the book bag by the door the night before
- Bringing completed homework and equipment back to school
- Keeping his papers tidy

Self-reliance also includes **time management**. Examples are:

- Starting homework without having to be reminded
- Starting homework the day it is set, rather than waiting until the night before it has to be turned in
- Planning realistically how long each piece of homework will take
- Not spending more time on homework than is needed so that he can have guilt-free downtime most days

- Completing homework before settling down in front of YouTube or Facebook
- Handing homework in on time
- Doing a bit every day on long-term projects
- Doing some daily and weekly revision, rather than leaving it until just before the quiz or exam

Self-reliance also has to do with 'real life'. We want children to be able to estimate realistically how long their activities usually take, such as homework, getting ready in the morning and travelling to school, so that they start to take responsibility for being on time. We want our children to be in bed early enough so they are getting enough sleep. We want them to not lose track of time in the morning so that they get out of the front door on time without a rush.

Self-reliance leads to self-confidence. This confidence comes from children being able to cope with their own lives, doing things for themselves, knowing that they are competent and knowing that their parents can trust them (most of the time) to do the right thing.

Within each of us there is a natural, very strong developmental drive to be autonomous, to make decisions for ourselves and to take care of our own lives. When too much is done for children, they are not exercising that natural urge and so they may drift into the habit of being powerful in other ways, such as getting attention by misbehaving or by seeming helpless.

And finally, school is much easier for children who are in the habit of self-reliance, especially secondary school. Having multiple teachers, multiple binders and textbooks and papers, keeping track of everything — this can feel like a nightmare for a child who is not prepared. And by the time a child reaches secondary school there are often penalties for forgetting to hand in homework or for handing it in late.

Why are some children and teens very self-reliant and others are not?

Environment is by far the most influential factor in determining how self-reliant a child or teen will be. This is good news because this is the factor parents can do the most to change.

A parent who is rushed or stressed often becomes impatient with the time it takes a child to do something on her own. This parent wants it done now, and of course it is quicker to do it oneself. Plus you know that it will be done properly. So it is tempting to keep doing something for your child even though you have a nagging feeling that your child really should be learning to do this for herself. This applies to homework-related tasks as well as to real-life tasks.

Interestingly, a parent who is naturally organised often produces a child who is very disorganised. The parent who cannot stand any mess may automatically jump in to do things for the child, instead of teaching and training the child to do it for himself.

When we start requiring our children to be self-reliant about some tasks, they soon develop competence and confidence in other areas as well. Going to the shops by themselves, giving their own order to the waiter, coming back from the shops with the right change, not only loading the dishwasher but switching it on, etc. — if we don't make sure children practise these tasks, they may come to believe that they are not capable. Or they may believe they should not have to do things because they have a live-in servant — you!

How can we guide children to become more self-reliant with their homework?

As parents and trainers, we need to remember that the purpose of homework is not just to get it done, although that may be what your children think. The purpose of homework is to learn something — not just to learn or revise the academic content, but, even more importantly, to learn more sensible, more mature, more self-reliant habits. Here is how we can teach and train self-reliance:

1 Slow down

Children need to be trained to be self-reliant and to develop enjoyable and productive homework habits. Habits can only become established over time; therefore training takes time. For us to be willing to make the time in our busy lives to train children in good habits we need to keep our focus on our long-term goals for our children. We need to think about what kind of people we are hoping they will grow up to be. It is easy to get sidetracked into short-term thinking, focusing on getting daily tasks over and done with as quickly as possible. Speed is the enemy of training. We need to slow down so that we can focus on leading by example. We need to make the time to demonstrate the actions that will lead to success with homework, such as looking words up in the dictionary for meaning and spelling, relaxing with a book, writing neatly and enjoying the challenge of learning new things.

2 Assume nothing!

Self-reliance is about getting into the habit of doing the right thing without having to be prompted. But before the habit of self-reliance can be trained, obviously the child needs to know how to do the task correctly without any subtle prompts or cues. Don't assume that your child knows how to do something, such as look up a word up in the dictionary, proofread and edit his work, do long division, revise, etc., until you have seen him do it on his own from beginning to end with no input from an adult.

3 Use think-throughs

An important strategy for improving self-reliance, including organisation and time management, is the *think-through*, which I explained in Chapter 6. Every time we do a one-minute *think-through* at a neutral time, asking our child to tell us what she should do and where and when and how, that habit becomes more established in the child's long-term memory.

4 Descriptively Praise

During the daily homework session and throughout the day, instead of telling or reminding, wait to see if your child remembers what to do and how to do it. Descriptively Praise whatever you can. That is often enough to motivate him to notice what he needs to do and how. But if not, give a little prompt, not a criticism or a lecture.

5 Do everything possible the evening before

We can guide children to be more organised by making sure that on school nights they do everything possible the evening before. In the evening there is more time to teach and train, whereas in the morning you may feel too rushed or preoccupied to take the time to make sure your children to do for themselves everything they are capable of doing for themselves.

In the evening, the homework needs to be packed away and the school bag by the door before your child's free time can begin.

6 Require your child or teen to organise himself every day

For example, train your child in the habit of always numbering the pages of his essays. If he needs to insert additional pages later, he can number them 1a, 1b, etc.

Also, require your child to use dividers in his binder between subjects and between topics within subjects.

KEY CONCEPT

Do not rescue your child!

Your child may forget to write down his homework or he may have written it down in a rushed, sketchy way so that when the time comes to do it he is confused. If the solution is to ring another child to clarify what the homework is, this is the child's job, not the parents' job. Your child may feel embarrassed about making the call or he may worry that he still will not understand what the instructions are. He may plead with you to make that phone call for him. If you do, you are unintentionally sending him the message that you will rescue him when he does not do his job, which is to come home knowing what his homework is. He is far more likely to learn this important lesson if he is the one who has to make the phone call.

How to teach and train more mature time management skills

Children who are disorganised often have only a very hazy idea of what their day or their week or their term looks like, in terms of their obligations. When we talk to our children and teens about when they should be where, it's often a matter of in one ear and out the other, even if they're paying attention. That's because information evaporates from the auditory short-term memory very quickly. Engage your child's visual strengths and you will see she remembers much more.

It helps to make a weekly timetable, which may change from week to week, so that everyone in the family can see at a glance when the after-school activities are and what time is available for homework, revision, music practice, household chores and playing. Making a timetable often shows everyone that they have been making some unrealistic assumptions. It is useful to make a weekly timetable even during the holidays because there will continue to be things the child has to do, such as revision, projects, exercise, etc.

Here is an activity you can do with young children all the way up to teenagers. With one child at a time, sit down in front of a big calendar, looking at this month or next month. Ask your child questions like those listed below. This will guide her to become much more aware of time.

How many Mondays are there in this month?
The last day of this month falls on what day of the week?
What date is the third Sunday of this month?
Which date is your science project due?
How many non-school days are there this month?
Which dates will you have your violin lessons on?
How many days in this month start with the letter T?

Which dates is Daddy out-of-town this month?
What day is the fifteenth of this month?
Which date is your Latin exam?
Does this month have an odd number of days or an even number of days?
How many days are there from today until your next football practice?
How many full weeks are there in this month?
What was the date a week ago?
Which day is Sam's party?
How many days until the weekend?
How many days until the weekend after next?
What special days are in this month?
What days of the week do those special days fall on?

CHAPTER 11

IMPROVING MEMORY AND GENERAL KNOWLEDGE

A few years ago when my daughter was thirteen, her maths teacher told us that she was really going to struggle with GCSE maths if she didn't start applying herself. My wife and I didn't really know what to do. How do you get a teenager to start applying herself? So we started sitting down next to her when she was doing her maths homework, and we saw how confused she was. Even basic things like fractions, she didn't seem to have a clue about. And then we discovered why. She didn't actually know her times tables properly. So she was guessing or trying to count up in her head or making lots of little marks on a piece of paper and getting herself all confused. So we made a family project out of Seema learning her multiplication tables. We did everything Noël says to do. We did the cumulative review, so she was revising all of them, not just one table at a time. We quizzed her in lots of different ways. She made flashcards so she could quiz herself. And we definitely did the overlearning. We didn't stop when she knew it. We kept going. At first, Seema was embarrassed to admit that she didn't know her tables. But pretty soon she got into it, and it was only five minutes a day so it didn't feel bad. My wife and I were amazed to see that as soon as she knew all her multiplication facts, everything else in maths got easier. It turned out that she wasn't rubbish at maths the way she thought she was; she was just missing one important building block.

Father of two teens, aged 15 and 13

Why memory matters

If your child does not easily remember the sorts of things that most other children of his age can easily remember, of course he will suffer academically. Many subjects require ongoing memorisation, for example:

- English — spelling, rules of punctuation, parts of speech
- Mathematics — bonds, multiplication facts, procedures
- Sciences — procedures, definitions, formulae
- History — dates, causes and effects
- Foreign languages — vocabulary, verb endings, idioms
- Other subjects — specialised terminology

In addition, your child may be less appealing as a friend if she is confused about what others her age take for granted. And she may have a harder time managing 'real life', including keeping track of her belongings and remembering when she needs to be where. Difficulties in these areas rapidly erode a child's self-esteem. These are very important reasons for actively helping your child to improve her memory.

Parents often express bewilderment that the same child who can't seem to remember to put a full stop at the end of a sentence can have such an excellent memory for topics that he is passionate about. Unfortunately, his 'specialist subject' is rarely a topic that will help him fulfil his academic potential. He may know, and want to tell you endlessly, all about every dinosaur ever discovered. Or he may be able to discuss knowledgeably the strengths and weaknesses of hundreds of Pokemon or Yu-Gi-Oh! creatures. Clearly this child has a well-functioning long-term memory for topics that sustain his interest.

So why does he have such difficulty remembering what we want him to remember? It is often because his short-term memory is relatively weak, immature, patchy and unreliable — and as yet untrained. Almost as soon as a piece of information enters his short-term memory, it starts to evaporate. This is especially true if he:

- Has relatively weak auditory processing, by which we mean that he cannot easily turn the words that are coming in through his ears into mental pictures that make sense as quickly as the teacher is talking
- Cannot yet read well enough to be able to take his attention off the process of decoding and put it on to the job of puzzling out the meaning of what he is reading
- Is a kinaesthetic learner, who becomes very restless and distractible when he is expected to sit still and absorb information passively
- Is emotionally under par because school is not a satisfying experience for him; he may be feeling anxious, embarrassed or resentful
- Is preoccupied with matters that seem far more important to him, such as who will play with him at break time or will his sandwich be soggy again today or will the teacher give him an annoyed look if he makes another mistake
- Already has some confusion about the topic and therefore does not quite understand what the teacher is talking about
- Is not interested in the topic in the first place

Short-term memory is the gateway into long-term memory. If a fact or concept or skill falls out of the short-term memory almost as soon as we put it in there, it is not staying in the brain long enough to be transferred into long-term storage. That is why a child can be told the same thing hundreds of times over many years, such as 'Start sentences with capital letters', 'Show your working out in maths', 'The word 'where' has an "h" in it', and still seem oblivious.

It should go without saying that it absolutely does not make sense to expect a child to memorise something before he understands it thoroughly. Proof of understanding is that your child can explain it to you:

- Correctly
- Without any subtle prompts
- In his own words
- Succinctly, without irrelevant or tangential additions

Parents assume that this first step, that of making sure the child understands the material, will happen at school. It should, but it may not. When this consistently fails to happen, parents need to take charge rather than letting the situation drift in the hope that it will soon improve. Let us assume for now that your child understands the material that he is expected to remember.

What often happens is that a child will conscientiously try to memorise this week's spellings, history dates or French vocabulary. Even when his efforts are successful, the information has only entered his short-term memory. Unfortunately for him, the next week a whole new set of facts needs to be memorised. Last week's facts, unless they are rigorously reinforced, will soon fade from his short-term memory. That is why a child can know his eight times table or his spellings perfectly one day and not know them a few days or a few weeks later.

The solution to this problem of rapid forgetting is to make sure that the information enters the long-term memory, from which it can be retrieved at will with minimal prompting, even after a long time has elapsed.

Micro-skills training

Micro-skills training is all about <u>accurate memory storage</u> of the small skills that make up any larger skill. We want the information or skills the child is practising to enter his brain in the correct form so that it can be retrieved in its correct form. For this reason, we want to prevent the child from 'practising' his mistakes.

Seven guiding principles follow that you can use to sharpen your child's short-term and long-term memory, leading to greater school success and increased confidence.

1 Cumulative review

One simple way for your child to transfer information into her long-term memory is to add an extra fifteen minutes to each day's homework session, whenever time permits. Choose three skills or topics you want your child to improve and spend five minutes a day on each, reviewing some of what was memorised in previous weeks. This is known as cumulative review.

Of course, five minutes a day will not be enough time to cover all the previously memorised material in any subject. But you will probably be amazed at just how much material your child can cover when you commit to this extra five minutes of review every day. That comes to thirty minutes a week or two hours a month or roughly five hours each term. That is more time than most children or teens spend reviewing past material, unless they are revising for a specific exam. Think how accurate and quick your child could become at his multiplication facts or spellings or French idioms if he were to practise this much! And five extra minutes a day on a topic or skill is practically painless.

I also recommend that you establish the habit of cumulative review at all weekends, half-terms and holidays, as well as on any days when the homework your child has been set does not take up the full homework hour.

2 Overlearning

Keep revisiting the material to be learned until your child can rattle it off correctly, quickly, fluently and with no prompts. Then revisit it some more! This is called overlearning, and it results in the information sinking into the long-term memory so deeply that your child will be able to recall and use most of it even under adverse circumstances, for example if he is tired, hungry, feeling unwell, overexcited or anxious.

The number of repetitions necessary for overlearning to take place is affected by numerous factors, both internal and external. When the material to be memorised is presented to the child through his strongest channels, he will absorb it more quickly and more thoroughly and he will be able to retrieve more of it more quickly. For most people, and this is especially true of most children who are experiencing school problems, the preferred cognitive channels are visual and kinaesthetic, that is, seeing and doing.

In addition, when a child is rested, relaxed, confident and engaged, his long-term memory stores and retrieves information more efficiently.

3 Association

We all memorise best, and we all retrieve best, when we can mentally attach a new fact to something we are already familiar with. All mnemonics work in this way. A mnemonic is a saying that helps us to recall information. For example, I can easily remember the fictitious name 'Roy G. Biv', and that gives me instant access to the colours of the rainbow in the correct order, which I certainly would not otherwise be able to reel off so fluently.

We can help our children to do the same thing. To start with, we can teach them to use all the mnemonics we already know, such as:

- i before e except after c . . .
- 30 days hath September . . .
- <u>Big</u> <u>e</u>lephants <u>c</u>an <u>a</u>lways <u>u</u>nderstand <u>s</u>mall <u>e</u>lephants (the first letters of this sentence spell *because*)

We can also make a project of asking friends and extended family to teach us their favourite mnemonics.

Although we may not be consciously aware of the process, many times every day we use the power of what we already know to help us access or work out things that we otherwise would find difficult or impossible to 'just remember'. We know and use many tricks to help us remember. Let's say that you are helping your child to memorise the five times table. He will find the process much easier if you teach him that the answers in the five times table always end in 0 or 5. This is something that we know but take for granted and rarely think about. But this fact will be very useful to your child as he is learning. Knowing this fact will help him to work out the right answer rather than impulsively blurt out his first guess. Later, when with repeated practice he is beginning to remember the answers, this important fact about the five times table will enable him to self-check his answers.

4 Metacognition

Metacognition is a word that has been coined quite recently. It is most often defined as 'thinking about thinking' or 'learning about how we learn'. When we guide our children to look for, notice and use aide-memoires and patterns, we are teaching them to think about how they think. Until recently, the assumption was that some people are good at learning (by which is usually meant understanding, remembering and using information or skills) and some people simply are not. We now know, thanks to a great deal of brain research, that our brains are extremely malleable and versatile, capable of learning how to learn.

One way we can help a child improve his ability to learn is to respond with a *diagnostic response* when he makes a mistake. A *diagnostic response* helps him to think about and understand why he made the mistake. Each time your child makes an impulsive or 'careless' mistake during memorising or during Stages One or Three of his homework (see Chapter 5), stop everything. Ask him to tell you what his mistake was and what he should have said or read or written instead. Give him a *diagnostic response* to help him to think about why he made the mistake.

For example, if you are helping your child to memorise the five times table, you might ask 'Five times five equals what?' and he might impulsively reply 'Ten'. Instead of saying 'No,' or 'Pay attention, for goodness sake!' or simply telling him the correct answer, a *diagnostic response* might be, 'Maybe you thought I said "plus" because 5 plus 5 makes 10. Plus is adding. But I didn't ask you to add just now. What are you practising?' Once he understands the reason for his error, you can help him to sharpen his auditory attention to detail by asking him both questions at random: '5 + 5? 5 x 5? 5 x 5? 5 + 5?'

Be willing to take the time to Reflectively Listen about his frustration or about his anxiety that he will never get it right or about his resentment of you for making him do something that feels emotionally uncomfortable.

5 Attempting to retrieve

For memorising to take place, it is not enough for the child simply to be exposed to the information, even if the exposure is very frequent. Think of all the bits of information that your child has heard or seen many, many times that have not yet sunk in. To be effective, the *cumulative review* must be active, not passive. In this context, 'active' means that the child needs to try to dredge up the information from his memory with fewer and fewer prompts. This is called 'attempting to retrieve'.

When we attempt to retrieve the same piece of information many times, it is as if the brain notices that certain information keeps being needed. The brain comes to the logical conclusion that this information must be very important. So the brain takes the sensible precaution of storing the information in the long-term memory, from which it can be accessed easily and reliably.

Something very interesting happens within the brain when we spend even a small amount of time, on a regular, frequent basis, attempting to retrieve previously learned material. The very act of attempting to retrieve seems to trigger the long-term memory into storing many related bits of information, even bits that we did not review.

Spelling is a typical example of this phenomenon. If you have your child practise spelling for just five minutes a day, within a few weeks his ability to spell many words that he has not even studied will improve significantly.

6 Repetition with variety

The more different ways a fact or skill is practised, the more solidly it will be embedded in the long-term memory. Different bits of the information will be stored in different areas of the brain. Some of those areas will probably be more efficient at remembering, which will lessen the negative impact of the less efficient areas. In addition, practising the information in several different ways will make it easier for your child to transfer the learning to new situations. For example, when a child must memorise history dates, he needs, at the very minimum, to be able to answer both of these questions: 'What year was the Great Fire of London?' as well as 'What happened in 1666?'

Of course, amongst the many different ways that he will practise any bit of information to be memorised, we must include whatever ways the child will need to reproduce the information at school. For example:

- In the weekly French dictation test, the teacher probably reads out each sentence only once or twice, in a conversational tone and relatively quickly. At the beginning of the week's revision, when your child is just becoming familiar with the new vocabulary, you will probably need to repeat each sentence or phrase very slowly several times, with exaggerated expression. But by the end of the week, he needs to be practising his dictation the way it will happen at school. Otherwise he will not be adequately prepared.
- For a child with an unreliable memory to do well on a written spelling test, by the end of the week he must be practising writing the words, not just spelling them aloud to you and not just using the letter tiles that I recommend in Chapter 18.

- Because one of the goals of spelling practice is for the child to spell correctly when he is composing essays and exam answers, he will need to practise his weekly spelling words by writing sentences. Otherwise, you may end up with a child who gets one hundred percent on the spelling test, but misspells those very words later the same day when he is writing a story.
- Going back to our questions about the Great Fire of London, the child needs to be able not only to say the answers, but also to write the information in full sentences that are correctly spelled, punctuated and capitalised. This takes practice!

7 Lengthening intervals

One more step is needed to achieve *overlearning*. As soon as your child can tell you the information correctly, quickly and fluently every day when you ask him, stop asking him every day and instead ask him every other day.

It may take him a few days or a week to regain the same speed and fluency as when you were asking him daily. Once he can recall the information easily when you are asking him every other day, move to asking him twice a week. Again, expect an initial drop in speed of recall and fluency. Once this has been re-established, ask for the information every week. When the response is quick and fluent again, ask every two weeks and then eventually every month for a few months. By then, the information will be securely locked in the long-term memory.

How to make memorising less painful and possibly even fun

Here are some important guidelines:

- Always keep the micro-skills and memorising sessions short — a maximum of five to ten minutes (even if your child pleads for more, which may well happen if you follow these guidelines rigorously).
- Always start with what you are sure your child knows. Easy questions first! This warms up his brain, as well as boosting his confidence.
- Each skill to be memorised needs to be broken down into bite-sized micro-skills.
- Always respond positively to every correct answer:
  - Smile
  - Descriptively Praise, eg
    - *I remember when you didn't know that.*
    - *You didn't rush. You thought about it carefully and your brain came up with the right answer.*
    - *Three correct answers in a row!*
  - Thumbs-up sign or other gesture of approval.
- Phrase your questions differently each time, such as:
  8 times 2 equals what?
  2 times 8 is what?
  What is the answer if you multiply 8 and 2 together?
  How many lots of 2 are there in 16?
  What times 8 makes 16?
  You may feel that you could not possibly dream up so many variations. With practice, however, you will surprise yourself.
- Establish some new routines by doing them consistently, such as:

- Number bonds for five minutes each time the family gets in the car
- French verbs for five minutes at dinner time
- Twenty correctly spelled words while waiting in the check-out line at the supermarket
- Six science facts before the bedtime story
- Five history dates while doing household chores together

● Guide your child to come up with a way he can remember a fact or skill more easily (see Association, earlier in this chapter).

● We need to recognise that anxiety often lurks beneath reluctance, resistance, arguing, complaining or rushing to get homework or revising over with as quickly as possible. We can address this anxiety with plenty of Descriptive Praise, Preparing for Success and Reflective Listening (see Chapter 6).

Improving auditory memory

Echo activity

This activity is appropriate starting at two or three years old and continuing all the way through the teen years. It will help your child improve her:

● Attention to auditory detail
● Accuracy, fluency and reaction time of auditory processing
● Ease of visualising what she hears
● Categorising skills
● Clarity of speech production

- Understanding of the difference between a phrase and a sentence
- Confidence

Remember to do this activity for no more than five or ten minutes at a time. Each time you do it, start at or near the beginning, even if your child mastered the first stages easily the last time. This will build confidence and ease him gently into the more difficult stages.

1 **Say 'Repeat after me' or words to that effect.**
Frequently vary the wording of your instructions so that your child's brain has to think a bit, rather than simply respond automatically. For example, you could phrase it like this:
Say this word.
Say this back to me.
Echo what you hear me say.

2 **If necessary, start at the very beginning stage by asking your child to repeat back to you single words.**
At first these should be short words, then longer words and eventually unfamiliar words.

3 **Once he can correctly repeat back to you single words, with no hesitation, have him repeat short phrases.**
For example, 'a small kitten', then longer and longer phrases, such as 'the small white dog with the loud bark'.

4 **Then have him echo complete sentences.**
At first these will be short sentences, then longer and longer sentences and finally sentences that include unfamiliar vocabulary.

5 **To improve your child's vocabulary, comprehension and fluency, have him practise paraphrasing each sentence in his own words.**

6 **Next, have him repeat back to you a series of separate words, either related (eg cat, dog, monkey, giraffe) or unrelated (eg school, horse, grass, square).**
   You may need to start with only three items in each series. But with frequent practice, your child's memory will improve, and he will eventually be able to hold four or five unrelated words in his short-term memory and an even larger number of words if they are related in some way and if he understands how they are related.

7 **To help your child learn to categorise more precisely, ask him whether the words in the series are related or unrelated.**
   If they are related, ask him to explain what those words have in common. When he tells you, require him to speak in full sentences.

8 **Then reverse the roles, so that your child takes a turn thinking up and saying the words, phrases, sentences and series of words for you to echo.**
   This step may be the most difficult for your child, but it is very important. Here your child is having to practise transferring what he has learned to a new and slightly more stressful context. This step will result in the most solid learning possible.

Learning 'by heart'

Every child will at various times in her school career be required to memorise poems, sayings, proverbs, prose passages, possibly a speech to be recited in assembly or a part in a school play.

Children with a history of underachievement often find these tasks frustrating, anxiety-producing and ultimately demoralising. However, memorising long passages does not have to be a soul-destroying experience for your child (or for you). It can in fact be something enjoyable that boosts his morale rather than tearing it down. To accomplish this you need to Prepare for Success before the school springs this task on him. You do this by training your child's brain in the skills needed for memorising long pieces.

Begin with rhyming poems of two to four lines. As your child's auditory memory improves, move on to longer poems.

Don'ts

1 Don't expect your child to know how to memorise before you teach him how.
2 Don't be annoyed or surprised by how quickly he forgets, by his confusion or by his reluctance to even try.

Dos

1 Before even asking your child to start learning the piece, make a point of repeating it aloud slowly, in a slightly louder than normal voice and with exaggerated expression, at least ten times. This first step is the most important, so do not rush it.

Do it at the beginning of every memorising session, even if you think it is no longer necessary. We must not underestimate how quickly children with auditory weaknesses can forget and how easily their already fragile self-confidence can be shaken.

2 Ask questions to make sure that your child knows the meaning of all words, phrases and idioms contained in the poem. As always, require him to answer in complete sentences, e.g. 'Clatter means a loud noise'.

3 The next step is the same as the first step, except that when you recite the poem you will omit the last word of each line, pausing expectantly as you smile at your child. For example:

> Old King Cole was a merry old . . .
> And a merry old soul was . . .
> He called for his pipe and he called for his . . .
> And he called for his fiddlers . . .

- If your child chimes in with the missing word, show that you are pleased. However, if after a pause of a few seconds at the end of each line he does not volunteer the missing word, then you simply say the word and carry on reciting until you reach the end of the next line, when you again omit the last word and wait expectantly for a few seconds for your child to provide it.

- This technique for eliciting a response is known as a *trailing statement*. It has a huge advantage over questioning a child, which is the traditional way of finding out if a child remembers something. Questioning can make an anxious or confused or resentful child even more unconfident, hesitant or rebellious. But with a *trailing statement*, the parent has not put the child on the spot. You have not asked him directly what the missing word is. So if he is not yet able to say it, he does not feel like a failure and he is not worrying about whether he is disappointing you.

- Carry on with Step 3 as many times as necessary until your child can confidently supply the last word of every line, with no prompts, hints or clues. In case you are concerned that your child might become bored, restless or frustrated, remember that he will be spending no more than five or ten minutes at a time on this activity.

4 When your child has mastered this, move on to omitting the last two words of each line and pausing for your child to supply the missing words.

5 Continue in this way, not rushing it, until he is reciting the whole poem. If you are willing to take this whole process as gradually as I am suggesting, your child's confidence will blossom. Soon he will start to get ahead of you, reciting more and more of the poem, not just the omitted words. Whenever that happens, give lots of Descriptive Praise, of course.

6 As soon as each verse of the poem is completely memorised, have him practise it:
    1. With expression
    2. With appropriate gestures and facial expressions
    3. Standing in front of a mirror
    4. Standing in front of family and friends
    5. By writing it in rough
    6. By writing it out neatly

7 Once your child can recite the poem perfectly, with no prompts, do not assume that your job is finished. The poem is not yet embedded in his long-term memory. *Overlearning* is needed, which is accomplished by *cumula-tive review* and by *attempts to retrieve* at *lengthening*

intervals. So several times a week, have your child recite some of his previously learned poems or prose passages.

Each month, add a new poem or prose passage or perhaps a carol or hymn he is singing at school.

It is well worth taking the time to help him understand and memorise the words. He will soon join in more and will become more interested and alert.

Improving general knowledge

Many underachieving children and teens have huge gaps in their general knowledge, not just in their knowledge of school subjects. Parents tend to accept their children as they are, and may not even notice these gaps. I frequently ask parents to jot down, over a period of a week or a month, all the information, not directly related to schoolwork, that they notice their child is confused about or oblivious to.

Here is a small sampling of information that children and teenagers with school problems or homework problems may have missed, taken from their parents' lists:

- Their complete address
- The full names, in the right order, of all family members
- The correct spelling of all the above
- The surnames of friends
- The full names of their school and their siblings' schools, including correct spelling
- What their relatives do for a living
- The home town of relatives they visit or write to
- The dates of Christmas, Hallowe'en and Guy Fawkes' Night
- The difference between a town, a city, a county, a country and a continent

- The names of major cities in England and other countries
- What was special about well-known historical figures
- Where their lungs are located
- What wheat is
- The characteristics of mammals
- That the moon orbits the Earth
- And in terms of life skills, how to operate a hoover, dishwasher, washing machine, microwave, etc. (at the appropriate ages)

Sometimes parents become defensive when I point out the gaps in their children's general knowledge, asking me, 'Why do these little facts matter?' This is a very important question.

These, and similar facts, are the foundation stones that children and teenagers need to have firmly in place in order to build a solid understanding of more complex academic subjects. Without this foundation of general knowledge, schoolwork, homework and real life will be far more confusing than they need to be. In addition, general knowledge adds immeasurably to a person's social skills, and people may regard him as odd if he is ignorant of commonly known facts.

And most importantly, knowledge of these and similar facts helps children to understand their surroundings, to feel comfortable and to respond appropriately. The more easily children can navigate their world, the more actively and the more successfully they will participate. The more often children can respond successfully, the more alert and aware they become. Their listening skills and their memory will improve. They will be more able to fulfil their potential in every area of their lives. All this leads to increased motivation, self-reliance and self-confidence.

Some of this general knowledge is no longer taught at school; some is taught but not systematically. Possibly the facts or concepts were taught several years ago, way back in infant school, often quite sketchily, during brief discussions that your child may not have been really tuning in to. Probably most of the children in his class mastered these facts and concepts easily, so the teacher's attention moved swiftly on to the next steps of the curriculum, leaving some children behind. So if you are committed to improving your child's general knowledge, you will need to teach him at home.

The technique known as *trailing statements*, which I explained earlier in this chapter, is very versatile and can be used whenever you want to help a child who may be impulsive, reluctant, immature, unconfident or anxious to understand or notice or remember something. For example, you might weave *trailing statements* such as these into your everyday conversations:

Next month is . . .?

The Prime Minister is . . .?

Today is Saturday, so the day after tomorrow is . . .?

Granny used to work in a shop, but now she's a . . .?

The sun is really a star, and the Earth is a . . .?

The Thames River runs through the city of . . .?

If your child does not respond within five or ten seconds, finish the statement yourself. Then immediately repeat the *trailing statement* for him to finish. When he can do this, have him say the complete sentence so that all the bits of information are stored together in his long-term memory.

CHAPTER 12

IMPROVING REVISION SKILLS

> My children used to complain whenever they had to revise for an exam, and I would naturally sympathise with them. I tried to make them feel better by telling them about how I hated to revise too when I was a kid, and my parents had to nag me constantly. I told them about a time when I hadn't revised Chemistry all year so I ended up staying up and revising all night the night before the final exam. My kids thought that was great and said they wanted to do that too. That was a wake-up call for me. I realised that my boys wanted to be like me so I had better be a good role model. Right then I completely changed tack. I had a meeting with each one, and we came up with a realistic revision timetable. Then I sat with them every night while they revised. That helped them to concentrate. I quizzed them every night, and they were so proud when they knew the answers. I gave them lots of Descriptive Praise for concentrating, for not complaining, for not giving up, for going over the same questions until they knew the answers. I took Noël's advice about using flashcards. They make revising so easy. My reward for all this effort came when the boys' attitude improved, and so did their marks. But what made me happiest was one day I heard them telling their uncle that revising was fun. That made me see that I was giving them a good habit for the rest of their lives.
>
> Father of three boys, aged 15, 14 and 9

When it comes to revising, most children, and especially teenagers, don't want to do it. And even if they are willing, do not expect them to want to revise <u>properly</u> or for <u>long enough</u>.

Parents often reinforce distaste for revision by allowing children to keep putting it off, while anxiety and guilt mount. In fact, there is nothing inherently unpleasant about revising. It can be a very enjoyable and satisfying activity. Our job is to teach our children how to revise effectively and enjoyably and to guide them into the habit of revising regularly. But expect resistance at first!

One form of resistance is questioning the usefulness or relevance of the information that they are supposed to be revising. Be warned: When you answer these questions by explaining why certain topics or skills have to be revised, your children and teens are not listening! So before you start explaining and justifying, recognise that every day at school your children do many things that they don't see the useful- ness of. They do those things without complaining because they are in the habit of doing them and because those things are not very difficult. But revising is difficult for children who have not been taught how or who have been allowed to leave the revising until right before an exam.

So don't get sucked into explaining. Your child is not listen- ing because the question 'Why do I have to?' is not really a question. It's usually just another way of saying he doesn't want to do it. And any pearls of wisdom that you might offer in explanation, your child has probably already heard. Instead, Reflectively Listen to the upset feelings that are lurking below the level of your children's complaints:

You look like you really wish you didn't have to revise tonight.

Maybe it just feels too hard.

Maybe you're worried that you'll revise for hours and you still won't do well on the exam.

Make sure to keep any discussion of why revision is necessary out of homework time and out of revision time. Afterwards, be willing to listen and to discuss. Interestingly, after the revision session is over, children and teens are usually not that keen to talk about why they have to revise. That is partly because, having done the revision, they are feeling the satisfaction that comes from completing something, especially something they were dreading. But another reason for not wanting to talk about it after they have finished is that questioning revision during revision time functions as a time-waster. Once the revision session is over, they don't want to use up their own time. They would rather be off playing.

Whenever you and your child or teen are discussing this important issue of relevance, rather than explaining to your child all the grown-up reasons why revision is useful, ask your child to take a sensible guess. If this is a discussion that he really wants to participate in, he will be willing to guess. If he answers 'I don't know,' or 'There is no good reason for revising,' then you can see that he is not really interested in thinking about this question.

This issue of the relevance or usefulness of revision usually fades away once parents undertake to make sure that children and teenagers know how to revise effectively and they are revising regularly.

How to revise

Do not expect your children, or even your teenagers, to know how to revise effectively. The purpose of revision is to memorise, to 'learn by heart'. What can be confusing is that the word 'learning' has two different meanings. One meaning is to understand, and the other meaning is to memorise. Those are two completely different stages. First comes understanding; then comes memorising.

A great deal has been written about how to revise. Most of these books have been written for GSCE or A level students on the assumption that by that stage young people are mature enough to motivate themselves to revise in the most effective way. Sadly, this is true for only a small minority of teenagers. Those revision tips and techniques are usually only useful if you and your child or teenager study them together and then you require him to practise them.

Children and teenagers often assume that all that is needed for revision is to re-read their notes. This is far too passive to be effective. During re-reading, the brain is not actively engaged in *attempting to retrieve*. So re-reading feels 'boring'. An added problem is that their notes may be incomplete or confused. If they wrote their notes in class, they probably did it in a hurry, resulting in messy and possibly illegible hand-writing. And when children re-read their notes, it all looks familiar so they assume that they know the information.

Make an index

To make revising less onerous, guide your child into the habit of making an index, similar to a table of contents, for the front of the binder that holds her revision notes. This will mean that she can easily and quickly find each subject, each topic and each sub-topic.

Make a list of key words

Require your child to make a list of the key words that he needs to understand and then memorise in each topic, along with their definitions and some examples. Compiling this list is actually the beginning of the revision process.

Use flashcards

In many research studies, flashcards have been proven to be the most effective way to memorise separate bits of information, such as the specialised terminology of each subject, foreign language vocabulary, multiplication facts, etc.

Do not assume that your child knows how to make flashcards or how to use them most effectively. The handwriting needs to be neat and the information on the cards needs to be boiled down to the essentials. Do not let your child copy verbatim from the textbook onto the flashcards. The words on the flashcards need to be in note form, short and succinct. In science, for example, you might have the name of a formula on one side and the formula on the other. For English, your child might write a word on one side and the definition (in her own words) on the other side. For foreign languages, she could write the English on one side and the translation on the other. Children often enjoy writing flashcards in different colours to signify different categories, and this is part of the revising process because their brain is already engaged in thinking about the material.

A very common mistake children make with flashcards is glancing at one side, assuming they don't know the answer and quickly turning the flashcard over to read the answer, before giving their brain time to attempt to retrieve the information. As I mentioned in Chapter 11, without *attempting to retrieve* the brain does not get the signal that this information is important enough to store in the long-term memory.

Here is a solution to this problem. At first use this method with your child to show him how. After a while he will be able to do this without your input. Lay out a number of flashcards on the table. Start with just a few at first so your child does not feel overwhelmed. Have him point to any flashcard he likes and tell you what is on the other side. Because the flashcards are laid out flat on the table, he cannot impulsively turn the card over in his hands, so he has to think about what is written on the other side.

You can introduce an element of friendly, non-threatening competition by keeping a tally of how many flashcards your child answers correctly. When you do the same activity the next day, he will be motivated to top his previous score. And he is likely to get a higher score because he is memorising the information. When your child is more confident, you can add a rule that the only answers that will count towards his score are answers that are correct the first time. This eliminates most impulsive blurting.

Revise daily

As I mentioned when explaining about *cumulative review*, children learn best when they revise a topic or subject or micro-skill every day, six days a week, rather than having a few marathon revising sessions right before exams. Daily revision results in information being stored in the long-term memory throughout the term. This reduces the amount of information that has to be memorised right before an exam. Plus, it helps the child to be successful throughout the term as he is building a solid foundation of facts and skills that are being embedded in his long-term memory.

Monitor the time spent revising

Research has shown that for maximum effectiveness, each revision session should be no more than forty to fifty minutes. Each revision period needs to be followed by a break. Make sure that the break is an active break to re-energise the brain.

A child or teen who is new to revision or who is very resistant may need to start with much shorter revision sessions, perhaps only fifteen or twenty minutes at a time. Day by day or week by week, you can increase the length of each revision session to build up your child's stamina for concentrating and for handling the uncomfortable feelings that often arise during revision.

The whole family needs to know at which hours revision will be happening and on which days. That way your child has much less 'wiggle room'. Have your child make a timetable, and then scrutinise it carefully to make sure it is realistic. It is quite common for children and teenagers to write on their timetable that they will be doing hours and hours of revision each day. They want to believe that they can force themselves to! They desperately want to do well, or perhaps they know they have left starting their revision until too late. But they forget that they dread revision and that when the time comes to revise, they will do everything they can to try and avoid it.

Your role in revision

Of course, parents want children to be able and willing to revise independently without the parents having to be involved. In order to achieve that goal, you will probably need to start by staying with them as they revise. The more enjoyable and productive you can make the revision activities, the sooner your child will feel confident to revise on his own. You may need to wean him off your presence in small steps. The first step might be that your child revises while you watch. The next step might be that you are sitting at the same table but doing your own 'homework', not watching your child. A further step might be that your child is revising while you are in the room but not sitting at the table with him. And eventually you will be in a different room and you will know that he is getting on with his revision without wasting time or complaining. That deserves a reward!

KEY CONCEPT

Quizzing your child

Children often want to be quizzed by a parent as a form of revision. This is partly because revising alone feels lonely, and whenever any of us has to do something that feels unpleasant, having company usually helps. Another reason that children prefer to be quizzed is that it is active and therefore more interesting. Parents tend to think that the quizzing should come after the child has revised for a while. But quizzing can usefully come first in order to discover what the child knows and what he doesn't know.

CHAPTER 13

IMPROVING THINKING SKILLS

> *I used to be very embarrassed because my son acted so childish. He acted as if he wasn't much older than his younger brother, especially at homework time, but actually he's six years older. Homework was a battle, trying to get him to work independently, and this was really frustrating me. My husband thought I was being too hard on him, and it used to cause rows between us. The school also said that he was immature for his age, wanting help from the teacher instead of think- ing for himself. So I decided to do something about it instead of just getting annoyed with him. I taught him how to do a lot of things for himself that I used to do for him, and whenever he acted like he couldn't do something, I always made him take a guess. I did lots of the thinking games with him because that gave him a lot of practice at problem-solving. Pretty soon he was doing better at school and was much more mature with homework and with his other responsi- bilities. In fact, now he sets a good example for his little brother.*
>
> Mother of two boys, aged 11 and 5

Thinking is what we do with our native intelligence. Thinking is making connections between what we know and what we don't know. Thinking is problem solving. Thinking is creating. Thinking is what is needed for school success and homework success.

The more we require children to use their brains, the more confident they will feel about using their brains. This seems obvious, but it is easy to forget that practice is needed to achieve progress and to achieve the confidence that comes with progress. Confidence in thinking enables children to do better work in every school subject and it also enables them to handle real-life problems more sensibly and maturely.

How parents can teach and train thinking skills

As with all the other school success skills, there are two ways that parents can teach and train thinking skills. One is within the context of homework and the other is outside of homework, in daily life, including through play.

Teaching and training thinking skills through homework

First, I am going to talk about how to use homework to improve thinking skills, and then I will describe some useful and enjoyable thinking games. You will see that many of the recommendations below have already been discussed in earlier chapters. That is because the teaching of thinking skills needs to permeate every aspect of homework.

1 **During the Stage One *think-throughs*, ask lots of *why* and *how* questions.**
   These questions challenge the brain the most.

2 **Don't do your child's thinking for her.**
   Assuming that the homework is not too difficult for her, she can always take a guess. And when children think they are just guessing, they are really *attempting to retrieve*.

3 **Don't allow your child to leave any blanks.**
Even if he feels stumped, he needs to write something down. This will stretch his mind.

4 **Require your child to answer you in full sentences during the Stage One *think-throughs* and to write in full sentences during Stage Two.**
This will sharpen his brain.

5 **Ask your child to paraphrase what he is reading.**
Do this not only with the text of his homework, but also with the instructions. This will guide him to think about what he is reading, and you will be able to notice and correct any inaccuracies or misconceptions.

6 **The *diagnostic response* in Stage Three, the improving stage, teaches your child about how her brain thinks (see Chapter 11).**
Once she is familiar with this process, start asking her to figure out for herself the *diagnostic responses* for her mistakes. For a spelling mistake you could ask 'Which two words did you mix up here?' For a sequencing mistake, you could ask 'Why would this be difficult for the teacher to understand?' For a factual mistake, you might ask 'How did you come up with this information?' As your child thinks about thinking, her thinking naturally improves.

7 **Descriptively Praise.**
Whenever your child shows evidence of mature thinking: speaking in full sentences, explaining things carefully, using more varied or more precise vocabulary, ordering his thoughts, etc., make sure you Descriptively Praise.

Teaching and training thinking skills through daily life, including play

Wherever we are and whatever we are doing, there are opportunities for us to guide our children to improve their thinking skills. Throughout the day there are many little problems that need to be solved: a mislaid shoe, a drawer that won't close, a machine that doesn't seem to work. As parents, we can solve these problems so quickly and so easily that the child barely realises there was a problem. Or we can involve children in the problem-solving process by asking leading questions and by taking the time to wait and listen while they fumble and experiment. This is how children learn, so this is what we need to do.

In addition, there are many enjoyable games that teach and train thinking skills and are especially good for the kind of 'guessing' that homework calls for. Some of these games require equipment, some require only a pencil and some paper, but many require no preparation or equipment at all. You can play these games at mealtimes, on family fun nights and whenever you and one of your children find yourselves with time to spare.

Deduction

This game teaches children the important skill of reasoning from evidence.

(a) One person writes down a question that he is sure no one in the group (including himself) knows the answer to. This step in itself challenges children to think.

(b) All the players write down their guesses about what the answer might be.

(c) Players discuss together which guesses are more sensible because the guesser used some knowledge and which are purely wild guesses.

An example might be the question 'What is the Prime Minister's middle name?' If one person guesses and writes down 'Jane', you can talk about the fact that a man is not likely to have a woman's name.

Categories

This game has an easier version, a more challenging version and an even more challenging version. Always start with the easiest. We want to build confidence by early success.

A Here is the easiest version:

(a) One person states a category. This could be a large category such as *food* or *animals*, or it could be a smaller category such as *farm animals* or *fruit*. It could be *means of transportation*, *countries*, *furniture*, *musical instruments*, etc.

(b) Everyone writes down items that belong in that category. Confident children may enjoy being timed to see how many they can produce in, say, five minutes. But an unconfident child is likely to feel anxious if timed, which would spoil her enjoyment of the game.

(c) If someone is stuck, another person can give a clue, such as the first letter or sound, the size or shape or colour, where this item might be found or how it is used, etc.

(d) Everyone takes turns reading out their items.

(e) Players discuss together whether all the items do fall into that category.

B In the more challenging version of this game, each participant tries to write down at least one item in the chosen category for every letter of the alphabet.

C An even more challenging version of this game is the same as B, except that together the players choose one of the items mentioned to represent each letter of the alphabet. Then each player has to repeat, in alphabetical order, all of the items. If your child is not confident that he can remember twenty-six items for the twenty-six letters of the alphabet, go from A to G the first time you play this game. The next time you play you can go from A to M and stop there. Each time you play, your child's memory and confidence will improve.

Type of what?

This is also a classification game. It reverses the thinking process needed for the previous game and it is more challenging.

A Here is the easiest version of the game:
(a) One person writes down a noun in a sentence that goes like this: 'An apple is a type of what?'
(b) The other players write down what categories that item could fit into. They could write 'An apple is a type of fruit' or 'An apple is a type of roundish food' or 'An apple is a type of food that can be baked in pies' (or sweet food or food that grows on trees or crunchy food etc.).
(c) Players discuss together the accuracy of the answers and which categories are wide and which are narrow.

B A more challenging version of this game is similar to A except that each player needs to write an additional item that also fits into the category they chose. So, someone might write, 'An apple is a type of roundish food, like grapes' or 'An apple is a type of crunchy food, like celery.'

Here's the answer so what's the question?

This game is the opposite of what usually happens in a classroom, where teachers ask questions and children are expected to know the answers.

(a) One person writes and then reads out an 'answer', such as *The Olympics* or *Seven* or *Under the bed* or *Swimming* or *Yes*. These 'answers' can be creative or silly.

(b) Each player writes down a question that would fit with that answer. If your child is unconfident or resistant or very young, require only one question. Over time, you will be able to require more and more questions.

Here are some examples of questions that would go with some of these answers. For the answer *The Olympics*, the questions could be 'What happened in London in 2012?' or 'What happened in ancient Greece every four years?' or 'Where do athletes from all over the world compete?'

For the answer *Seven*, players might contribute the questions 'How many days are there in a week?' or 'What number is four more than three?' or 'How many dwarves did Snow White make friends with?'

For the answer *Under the bed*, the questions might be 'Where do some people keep their bedroom slippers?' or 'Where do you often find a lot of dust?' or 'Where does a frightened cat like to hide?'

Mismatch

This thinking game sharpens children's understanding of categories and teaches them how to observe and explain similarities and differences.

(a) One person writes down four words. Three of the words will belong in the same category, and one of the words will not, for example:

Shop, bank, apple, library
Person, elbow, neck, foot

Huge, enormous, terrible, gigantic

Dog, tiger, cat, guinea pig

(b) All the players write down what the category is that three of the words fit into and which word does not fit into that category.

(c) Players discuss together what the category is and why each word does or does not fit into that category.

One hundred uses

This game awakens children's creativity and sharpens problem-solving skills.

(a) One person writes down the name of a familiar object, such as a cup, pencil, pillow, hat, ladder, piece of paper, light bulb, etc.

(b) Everyone writes down possible uses for that item. For *cup* players might write:

A holder for small objects such as coins or stamps

A biscuit cutter

A trap for a spider

An object to draw to practise perspective

(c) Players discuss together whether the item could really be used in that way. Accept all reasonable responses and ask for a further explanation if you don't understand the reasoning behind an answer.

Fact, fiction or opinion

This game teaches children to think carefully about what they hear and read.

(a) One person writes down a sentence and reads it aloud. For example:

Deserts are dry places.

Camping is fun.

Scotland is an island.

(b) All the players write whether they think the statement is fact (definitely true), fiction (definitely not true) or opinion (a personal belief that is not necessarily true).

(c) Each player explains his or her reason. You may be surprised by some of the reasons. This activity will show you what your child knows (facts vs fiction) and how they reason. As you correct any incorrect answers, your child is learning more about thinking.

Variation: For a very unconfident child who may not believe he can compose his own statements, the parent can write the sentences at first. After playing this game a few times, your child will grow in confidence and will become willing to make up his own statements.

How are these alike?

This thinking game teaches children to look for and understand similarities and differences, a very important skill.

(a) One person writes down two nouns and reads them aloud.

(b) All the players write down ways in which these two items are similar. For example, if someone writes down *sweater* and *blanket*, the sentences that describe the similarities might be:

> *They are both used to keep warm.*
> *They both are used by people.*
> *They both cover a person.*

If someone wrote down the two nouns *fish* and *soap*, you might get sentences such as:

> *They both can float.*
> *They both go in water.*
> *They both are slippery when they're wet.*

(c) Players discuss together whether the statements are accurate.

Connections

This activity helps children think outside of the box.

(a) Each player writes down several nouns that they think are interesting. Aim for a total of about ten words altogether.

(b) Everyone then writes down all the other players' words, so that everyone ends up with a list of exactly the same words.

(c) Each player thinks about, and writes down, any connections he can find amongst the listed words. For example: if the list consisted of these words: *elbows, rhinoceros, gum, Christmas, biscuits, film, cloud, scooter, font* and *clock*, some of the sentences might be:

> *A rhinoceros has elbows.*
>
> *You can chew gum while watching a film.*
>
> *I got a scooter for Christmas.*
>
> *You could look at a clock to see if the film is about to begin.*
>
> *People eat fancy biscuits at Christmas.*

(d) Players take turns reading aloud their sentences.

(e) Players discuss together whether the connecting ideas make sense. Accept all reasonable explanations.

How many questions?

This game guides children to think deeply and carefully about things they are used to taking for granted.

(a) One person thinks of a familiar object such as a house, a book, a table, etc., writes it down and announces it to everyone.

(b) All the players write down as many questions as they can think of about that object. For example:

> *What colour is it?*
>
> *What shape is it?*
>
> *What is it made of?*
>
> *How was it made?*
>
> *Who made it?*

Has it ever been repaired?
Can it be recycled?
Is it new or old?
How long will it last?
What is it worth?
What shop sells it?
How could it be improved?

(c) Players read their questions aloud and together discuss how they could find out the answers. Also discuss whether any of the questions are asking the same thing, but using different words.

(d) Each player chooses two questions that someone else contributed and makes up and writes down the answers to those questions.

(e) Players discuss together how accurate the answers are. For any answer that is incorrect or incomplete, discuss together how to improve that answer until the whole group is satisfied.

SECTION FOUR

LITERACY: THE FOUNDATION
OF SCHOOL SUCCESS

CHAPTER 14

IMPROVING LISTENING SKILLS

My husband and I have always thought of our kids as bright and intelligent, but their schools didn't seem to have the same opinion of them. One reason was that they left their homework until the last minute and then rushed through it, doing the bare minimum. It was frustrating, but it was also embarrassing. We've got five children, so I have to admit, life was pretty chaotic and overwhelming. Even after I read about Preparing for Success and micro-skills, I just didn't have the energy to really do it. I did a bit of Descriptive Praise and a bit of Reflective Listening. It helped them to bicker less, but homework was still a nightmare. The final straw came when my youngest child's teacher said maybe he should be tested for ADHD because he just wasn't concentrating or getting on with his work. I didn't want him to be labelled and medicated so I thought, let's see what we can do by using Noël's strategies. So we immediately started with the Preparing for Success. We did lots of think-throughs about each subject until we were sure that all the children understood what their teachers expected from them. We practised keeping our voices friendly so that they would want to listen to us. We said a whole lot less, but we meant what we said. We even spoke in short sentences. Amazingly, all five of our children improved a lot from this. They started cooperating much, much more than before. And homework went so much more smoothly. Pretty soon their school reports were much better, and we could see that they were really starting to feel good about themselves. It was such a relief. Now we know they're intelligent, and so does the school.

Mother of five children, aged 21, 19, 16, 13 and 12

We think of school as being mostly about reading and writing. But studies have shown that between eighty and ninety percent of what a student is supposed to be doing in the classroom is listening. This is as true in secondary school as it is in primary school. They may be listening to instructions about work or behaviour, which they are then expected to remember and follow. They may be listening to information about subject matter, which they will be expected to remember and then demonstrate an understanding of, usually by writing. So we can see how disadvantaged any pupil will be if he has even mild problems with any aspect of auditory processing,

Fortunately, listening is a skill that can be taught and trained. Listening is about paying attention and is a function of the brain, whereas hearing is a function of the ears. When we listen our brains are active:

- Without thinking about it consciously, we choose which sounds to pay attention to and which sounds to tune out as irrelevant. Only then can we comprehend. But this skill is often weak in children who are not fulfilling their potential.
- Once our brains decide which sounds we should be paying attention to, then we need to discriminate between similar sounds.
- Our brains make sense of what we hear by connecting it to something we already know. If this sequence of events is not happening reliably, both listening comprehension and reading comprehension will remain patchy and immature. If a child does not fully understand the sentences he hears, how can we possibly hope that he will understand these same sentences when he reads them, even if he is able to decode them accurately?
- We store the important information in the right order, first in our short-term memory.

- Eventually, with accurate repetition, the correct information is transferred to our long-term memory (see Chapter 11).

Auditory processing weakness is hard-wired into the brain, long before birth. So as parents we continually have to keep two aims in mind:

- First, we need to 'work around' the child's processing difficulties so that he can access the curriculum without being handicapped by his cognitive weakness.
- Second, we need to help this child improve his receptive language skills, by which I mean his ability to understand what he hears, so that he can function more and more independently and maturely. Luckily, the brain is extremely malleable, so the areas of weak functioning can be strengthened considerably. As he learns to understand what he hears better, he will automatically be learning to understand what he reads better.

Techniques to help your child learn to listen better

Some of the following techniques to help your child learn to listen better function as crutches — they simplify or slow down the stream of language that is coming into the child's brain. This will give him a better chance of understanding what he hears. Other strategies are designed to strengthen his listening skills. Some of the strategies accomplish both aims.

- Avoid calling your child's name to get her attention. Children hear their names being called many, many times, too often uttered in an irritated tone of voice. Children may assume something not very pleasant is coming when they hear their name so they don't want to pay attention.

- Make it a firm habit to give and get eye contact before you even begin speaking to your child, whether you are asking, telling or answering.
- Keep your voice low. It can be as difficult for your child to understand you when you bellow as when you talk too softly.
- Keep your voice friendly, calm and enthusiastic. No child will be motivated to listen to a tone that is abrupt, impatient or irritated.
- Speak more slowly than usual, with longer pauses between sentences and also longer pauses between the phrases within each sentence. This is how we automatically speak to young children because we know that they cannot make sense of a long stream of words. The child with poor auditory processing is still at an immature level, so he still needs this from us.
- Make a point of articulating very clearly.
- Speak in short, simple sentences. Put each new piece of information into a new sentence. This will help your child to visualise what he hears.
- Finish your sentences. Once you start listening carefully to yourself and to others, you will see how common it is for people to say the first few words of a sentence, not finish that thought, and then start a new sentence.
- Completely finish each thought before you go on to the next point you want to make. This will cut down on confusion.

Improving listening during homework time

Before you launch into the details of what you want your child to do, Prepare for Success by giving him one or two summary sentences as an introduction. This wakes up the child's brain and alerts him to what he should pay attention to, i.e. what to visualise. Avoid overloading his weak auditory processing with a stream of sentences, for example:

Where's your homework diary? I need to see what spellings you've got this week. I hope you copied them down properly. Last week you got eight out of ten right. Do you think you can do even better this week?

This is too much information coming at him too quickly. It is too great a processing load for a child with an auditory processing weakness. He will feel swamped, even though he is perfectly capable of understanding each sentence if he is given enough time to digest it before the next one comes at him.

When a child reacts to the river of words by arguing or complaining or trying to change the subject, parents may assume, often incorrectly, that the problem lies with the subject matter or with the teacher or with the school. There may indeed be problems in those areas, but often the underlying problem is that the child cannot translate the words he hears into mental images as quickly as the other person is talking.

It is more helpful to introduce the homework very simply, by saying something like 'Now it's time to practise your spellings'. Then stop talking and wait for a response. Your child may just sit there motionless, looking at you blankly, or he might be staring off into space. You may be wondering whether he is ignoring you or being deliberately disrespectful or maybe he simply didn't hear you. But as long as you remember to talk to your child only when he is looking at you, you will know that he has heard you. After long seconds have elapsed, he may eventually begin searching for his spelling list, in which case you can Descriptively Praise: 'You're getting started even before I told you to. That's self-reliance (or responsibility or courage, etc.).' Or he may complain or argue. That is your cue to Reflectively Listen: 'You probably wish you were a naturally good speller!' or 'Maybe you're worried that you'll make lots of mistakes and I'll get annoyed.' Then wait for him to respond.

Do not repeat yourself!

There may be many occasions during the daily homework session when you will feel tempted to repeat your instruction, for example if he was not listening the first time you said something or if he seems confused or if he impulsively makes the same mistake again and again.

Don't repeat yourself! If you do, your child's brain will not get the message that he needs to listen. Here is what to do instead:

- Before you start speaking, wait and make sure that he is looking at you. If he looks away or starts fiddling while you are talking, pause and wait for his attention.
- Keep explanations short. After two sentences, you have probably lost his attention.
- Keep him focused by pausing after every two or three sentences and asking him to tell you what you just said. Do not move on to your next point until he can tell you in his own words. That is how you can be certain that he has not only heard, but understood.
- Get into the habit of repeating and emphasising key words when you are explaining. These repetitions will help his brain sort the incoming information more efficiently.
- Challenge yourself to use more concrete and vivid vocabulary, which will help your child construct a clearer mental picture.

CHAPTER 15

IMPROVING READING: ACCURACY AND FLUENCY

My five-year-old is the oldest of four. I used to feel very guilty because I never seemed to have any time to play with her or even to listen to her read. And she wasn't good at reading so she kept hiding her book or saying that she didn't know how to sound things out. I didn't want her to feel bad about herself, so I was determined to take the time to help her practise. I put the other children to bed earlier, and I started listening to her read at bedtime, but then I read where Noël says that that's not a good time because the child's brain is tired by then, so I did something very drastic. For twenty minutes every day, I put the younger three kids in one room with plenty of toys and I left them there, even if they were crying. And I spent the twenty minutes just concentrating on Hallie, my older daughter. I realised that she didn't really know the alphabet properly, so I taught her that. She didn't know all her sounds, so I taught her that next. We played the Matching Game, the Scrambled Sentences, the Rhyming Tennis and I taught her how to sound out the first three letters of every word. One of the things she really liked about our reading lessons was that I put the other three in the other room and they couldn't come out. That really impressed her and showed her that I just wanted to be with her. Her reading got better every day, and by the end of the term, she was one of the best readers in the class. I almost stopped then, but we kept going with the little reading lessons because they're a lot of fun for both of us, and it's a time when I can just concentrate on her. And the other three very quickly got used to playing by themselves without my attention so I don't have to feel guilty about that.

Mother of four, aged 5, 3, 2 and 8 months

When we say that children have learned to read we mean several different things. We mean that they can quickly and accurately decode even unfamiliar words that are mostly phonetically regular or that follow a known spelling pattern (such as silent 'e').

We also mean that they can read by sight, without having to decode, many small, phonetically irregular words because they have read them correctly so many times that their brain now knows those words. For example, when they see the word 'come' they know that it does not rhyme with 'home'.

We also mean that they remember how to read phonetically irregular words that they have encountered several times in their reading.

When they are reading aloud we expect children to glide the words together, so that the sentences sound natural, as if someone is talking rather than reading word by word, which sounds stilted. This is known as fluency. Even when a child does not yet read with very good expression, we do expect the child to stop at the end of a sentence, to pause slightly when he comes to a comma and to make his voice go up when there is a question mark. In this chapter I will explain how parents can improve the accuracy and fluency of a child's reading.

We also expect that children will understand what they are reading. In the next chapter I talk about how parents can improve reading comprehension.

You can use the recommendations in this chapter to supplement the school's teaching if your child is not making the progress with reading that you would like.

Activities to improve the accuracy and fluency of your child's reading

It is never too early or too late to become a good reader. You can use the activities in this section to give your child a head start or to help a child who has fallen behind. This can be particularly useful if you have a child who is very sensitive or easily distracted or who tends to be anxious. This child may become distracted or disturbed in a busy, possibly noisy classroom, full of sights and sounds that grab his attention. Such a child may not be able to concentrate well enough at school to learn what he should be learning, even though he is perfectly capable of learning in a quieter, calmer environment.

You may have a child who needs more repetition than others in order to embed a concept or skill in his long-term memory. If he is left to practise on his own, as often happens in the classroom, he may be practising his mistakes (if he is paying attention at all). At home, you can supervise the reading activities so that most of the time error-free learning is taking place. That way you will know that the correct information is going into his long-term memory.

Do not feel that you need to work with your child in the same way that the school is teaching reading. Sadly, many teachers are far too busy labouring at the chalk face to keep up with all the new research being published in educational journals on improved ways to teach reading. Also, the more different ways a child learns something, the more parts of his brain are engaged, and the greater likelihood there is that concepts and skills will be understood and remembered.

You may be concerned that a young child might be too restless to sustain concentration on the following activities. He may complain or walk away or say, 'It's boring'. Parents often conclude from these behaviours that the child is simply not interested in learning to read or is too immature and not ready to learn. In fact, the child's negative reaction is much more likely to be because the activity is unfamiliar or because the parent is expecting the child to concentrate for too long or because the parent is expecting the child to remember something before he has had adequate repetition. The solutions to these problems are:

- Set a timer for five minutes and put the timer out of reach so that your child will not be distracted by it. Be prepared to stop the activity in mid-flow when the timer goes 'ding'. This way your child will soon trust you that five minutes of something he is not looking forward to really is only five minutes.
- Descriptively Praise all tiny improvements and all nearly right answers.
- Don't ask questions as this often makes an unconfident child go blank from anxiety. Instead, use the *trailing statements* I explained in Chapter 11.

Matching game

Choose three or four words that you think your child should be able to read but that he still finds problematic. Write each word on a separate piece of card. Then make a matching set of the same words. As your child matches the pairs he is learning to look carefully at the letters in each word. When that becomes too easy, add more pairs, including words that differ by only one letter, such as *pin* and *pen*. A more advanced version of this matching activity is to write the words to be matched in different sizes or colours or fonts. You can move on to writing one word in print and its pair in joined-up writing.

Sound sorting

This activity helps children differentiate between sounds that they may find confusing, such as *short i* as in *pig* and the *short e* sound as in *peg*. Looking through magazines, together cut out words with those sounds or pictures of objects with those sounds. Have the child put the *short i* words or pictures in one pile and the *short e* words or pictures in another. Then mix both piles together and have your child sort them into the two correct piles again.

Scrambled sentences

With word tiles, which can be bought or made out of card, have your child make a sentence that she can read easily. Together add words to make the sentence longer, more interesting and more challenging. When your child is able to read the longer sentence correctly, mix up the word tiles. Your child then unscrambles the sentence by putting the word tiles in the right order to remake the original sentence. In order to do this she has to focus on reading the individual words, whereas earlier she may have been parroting the sentence from memory.

Rhyming tennis

In this game the participants are 'batting' rhymes back and forth. One person starts the game by saying a one-syllable word, for example *tree*. Going around a circle, or going back and forth if only two people are playing, the next person says a word that rhymes with the first. Continue batting the same rhyme back and forth until your child cannot think of any more rhymes for the original word. At that point the parent can give some clues for additional words. Then the parent or child writes down as many of the rhymes as everyone can remember. Together talk about which words have a similar spelling (*see, tree*) and which do not (*me, Brie*).

Find and circle

This next activity is very versatile. You can use it to teach a child who is confused about any aspect of starting to read. Using old magazines or newspapers, have your child circle or highlight:

- Upper-case or lower-case letters (this will familiarise your child with the basic shape of each letter, even though the shape may possibly be distorted by a font he is unfamiliar with)
- Sight words, such as *the, they, their, there*
- *Silent e* words
- Three-letter words
- Categories of words, such as proper nouns, animals, colours, etc.

Singing helps reading

Choose a song your child knows well. Write the words (very neatly, of course, as we want to set a good example) and sing the song as you point to the words. Have your child join in with the singing and the pointing. Most songs have rhymes at the end of each line. This activity will guide children to see that the same letters usually make the same sounds in different words.

How to help children get the most from the reading books they bring home from school

The following guidelines will bring your children's reading books to life. Your children will see that books matter to you and are an important part of daily life. They will absorb your enthusiasm and that will motivate them to keep reading and learning.

- Read the books yourself so that you can talk about the characters and the events.
- Wonder aloud about what will happen next or why a certain character did what he did.
- Ask your child to quiz you to see if you remember what happened in the story.
- Bring the books into daily conversation:

That little girl looks like Chip.

Wouldn't it be fun if animals could talk like Paddington?

We could go to the Natural History Museum, just like the brothers did in your book.

- When you ask your child questions about her book, avoid questions that have a *yes* or *no* answer because those do not prompt her brain to do much thinking.

What to do when your child is stuck on a word

There are two schools of thought about how children should be helped when they get stuck on a word while they are reading. One approach focuses on the context, guiding the child to find clues in the picture or to think about what has happened already in the story and to make a connection or a prediction. The other method focuses on phonics, teaching children to sound out the word. Most teachers realise that this is a false controversy because both approaches are helpful.

When a child is reading and gets stuck on a word or misreads it, I recommend that you start with the context approach. You can ask a few questions to guide your child to think about what would make sense in the story. And that is often enough for the child to read the word correctly.

If that does not do the trick, then move on to the phonics approach. But the usual way this is done is not the most effective way. The usual way is to have the child sound out all the letters in the word, with the assumption that he will then be able to blend those letters into a word. However, even if the word is phonetically regular, this approach often causes problems because by the time he sounds out the last letters in the word, he may already have forgotten the beginning sounds. Another problem is that the usual sounds are not always a good clue to how the word is pronounced. It is not uncommon for beginning readers to sound out, 'T - I - M - E,' and say, 'Timmy,' or sound out, 'K - I - S - S,' and then say, 'cuddle!'

If the print in the book is quite small, I recommend that you write out the word (neatly, of course) on a blank piece of paper in larger print, which will be easier for your child's brain to process. Then cover up all of the word except for the first three letters. Have your child blend together those first three letters and guide him to think about which word that makes sense in the story starts with those sounds. That is often enough for the child to work out the word.

Careless mistakes

Readers of all ages and all skill levels sometimes read *a* for *the,* or *into* for *in,* or even *road* for *street.* This is not a problem if it happens only occasionally. But some children do this a lot. What is going on in the brain when this happens is very interesting. At the moment when they are saying *in* for *on,* they are not actually reading. Although their eyes may be resting on the word, the message from their eyes is not being relayed to the part of the brain that processes reading. A different part of the brain is operating, the part that uses context to guess at the next word (very similar to the 'predictive text' that is used on mobile phones). What is happening is called *psycho-linguistic guessing*. The child's brain is supplying a word that would fit the context, but the child is not actually decoding.

Most teachers and most books about reading recommend that parents not correct this type of mistake as long as the basic meaning of the sentence is not changed. I disagree. Children need to learn to read accurately, to read the words that are actually on the page. Professionals suggest not to correct these little mistakes because they worry it will interrupt the flow of the story, spoiling the child's enjoyment of reading. Also, they are concerned that parents may correct in an impatient, irritated way, which can undermine the child's confidence and his enthusiasm for reading. But teaching children to read accurately does not have to be done in a way that feels bad to the child.

Rather than having your child read to you in the usual way, start by explaining that you and she will each read alternating sentences. Introduce a rule that each sentence must be read correctly before the next person can start reading their sentence. That way, if your child makes a mistake when reading her sentence, you don't need to say anything. Just wait and don't start reading your sentence yet. That will give your child a clue that she made a mistake and needs to re-read her sentence. Model a positive attitude by being willing to re-read your own sentence after even a very minor stumble or mistake. Because children would rather not repeat their sentences, they very soon start paying attention to reading each word carefully. And this is accomplished with absolutely no impatience or telling off.

Teaching children to read words made up of several syllables

Most children eventually become quite skilled at reading the familiar words in their school reading schemes. These are mainly one-syllable words. But making the leap from reading those smaller words to reading longer words is often problematic. The child is likely to glance at the word, realise that he doesn't recognise it and take a guess, usually based on the first letter and on the context of the sentence. The word the child guesses is often incorrect. And even if his guess happens to be correct, he did not actually decode it so he may be just as perplexed the next time he comes across that word in a different context.

The following series of steps teaches children how to decode polysyllabic words. Start with two-syllable words, and then gradually build up to longer and longer words.

1   Choose several two-syllable words by browsing through the books you regularly read to your child. Choose words that she understands the meaning of, but does not yet know how to read reliably, such as *happy, problem, singing*.

2   Write each word on a piece of card, and cut the word in two at the syllable break. Do this with your child watching and, as you cut, point out that most of the time the next syllable starts with a consonant. So you would separate the words above like this: *prob / lem, hap / py*. Endings like *ed* and *ing*, which are separate syllables, are an exception to that rule. So *singing* would be divided like this: *sing / ing*.

3   Put the two pieces of card that make each word together on the table and read each word aloud as you point to it.

4 Have your child point to each word and echo what you just said.

5 Cover the second syllable and read the first syllable aloud, as you point. Then cover the first syllable and read the second syllable aloud, as you point.

6 Now have your child read each syllable separately as you just did. She may find this difficult at first because most of the syllables will be non-words (*prob, py, ing*) so she cannot match what she is reading to an image in her head.

7 Then mix up all of the syllable tiles on the table in front of your child. Her job is to put the right pairs of syllables together to make the words and then to read them.

8 The next time you do this activity, which should be no more than two days later, use the same two-syllable words. You may find that your child can read the syllables with no difficulty, or you may find that she has forgotten some or most of what she practised in the previous session. This time it won't take her as long to master reading the separate syllables.

9 Once she can read these syllables easily, add a few more two-syllable words, cut up into syllables, and mix them in with the earlier words. This will stretch your child's cognitive capacity.

10 You can be teaching your child to spell these syllables at the same time as she is learning to read the syllables. Have her look at a syllable and say the letters, then close her eyes and imagine seeing those letters in her mind. Then have her say the letters that she 'sees'. In Chapter 18, I talk more about how to guide children to become competent and confident spellers.

Improving reading fluency

When children start reading, they are decoding word by word, which often results in a staccato rhythm that sounds a bit like a robot might talk. This stilted way of reading can become a habit.

We want reading to sound natural, as if someone is talking. If this is a problem for your child, here's an activity that will teach her to read with fluency.

1   Choose a book that you know she can read without too much of a struggle.
2   Read a few sentences aloud as she moves her finger along underneath the words. This will ensure that she is reading as she listens rather than simply listening. Read with slightly exaggerated expression so that she can easily understand the meaning you want to convey.
3   Next, have her re-read the same sentences, copying your pacing and expression. She may be resistant at first, assuming it will be too difficult. Do insist, with lots of Descriptive Praise and Reflective Listening, because this activity will help her get into the habit of reading with fluency.

The importance of reading aloud

Read to your child every day, long past the age when he is capable of reading to himself. For children to do well at their schoolwork and homework, they need to continually hear more mature vocabulary and sentence construction than they are exposed to in the books they might choose to read to themselves. If your child is extremely restless and fidgety, he may find sitting still and listening to you read 'boring'. So read to him while he is playing with his blocks or Lego. In addition to bedtimes, mealtimes present another ideal opportunity to read to children. For more about reading aloud to your child, see Chapter 16.

Show your child that reading is everywhere

Wherever you are, point out words. At home, point out words on food tins and packets, and talk about the information those words give us. Direct your child's attention to interesting pictures in newspapers and magazines and read the captions that accompany them. Point out the titles of television programmes. You can even make labels for objects in your house.

Outside, point out street signs, street names, advertising posters, place names on public transport, words in shop windows. Point out the messages on people's T-shirts, and talk about what they mean. Show children brochures for events and places that would interest them. Whenever there are words and pictures together, point out how the words relate to the pictures.

How to make books special, important and pleasurable

- Continue to read to your children long after they can read to themselves. Show your enthusiasm by talking about how much you are looking forward to reading to them.
- Keep your children's books in a special place, and make sure that the books are kept tidy and accessible.
- Take your children to the library regularly. Leave enough time so that they can browse without feeling rushed.

Beware that nowadays most libraries have computers and that your child may gravitate to them rather than looking at books. You can make a rule that your child doesn't go on the computer in the library.

- Take your child to bookshops, not only when you are planning to buy something, but just for the pleasure of browsing. Show an interest in whatever books your child is drawn to. Even children who are not particularly excited about books are likely to want you to buy them a book once they are in a bookshop. You can set things up so that your child has earned being bought a book, or you can establish a routine of buying your child a book once a fortnight or once a month. You may worry that this will become very expensive. Think of it as a wise investment rather than as an expense.
- Take your children to charity shops, which have very inexpensive children's books.
- In addition to re-reading stories that your child likes, you can retell familiar stories together, with each person contributing the next sentence.
- You can act out familiar stories together.
- Whatever you may privately think about comics, do not show disapproval as that is likely to make them even more appealing to your child. Listen politely for a few minutes if your child wants to tell you about them, but do not include them in your reading aloud time.

Boys and reading

Even when both parents work long hours outside the home, children tend to spend more time with their mothers than with their fathers. Mothers are the ones who usually supervise homework and who are more likely to go in to school to talk to the teacher. And most teachers are women. This can leave boys feeling that learning, and reading in particular, is something that females care about, but is not really that important for males.

To counteract this understandable, but erroneous, conclusion, boys need the involvement of fathers, stepfathers, grandfathers, uncles and older male cousins in their learning. The key is for male family members to openly show their pleasure and approval when boys are reading, regardless of whether the reading is going smoothly or is a struggle. Boys need to see adult males reading books (not just newspapers), recipes, menus, instruction manuals, etc. This will help boys to see that reading can be enjoyable and useful.

CHAPTER 16

IMPROVING READING: COMPREHENSION

> *My daughter's at university now, and it's hard for me to remember that we used to have a big problem with her not wanting to read because now her subject at uni is Literature. When she was thirteen, it all came to a head. It wasn't only that she didn't want to read for pleasure, which was so disappointing for her father and me, but she didn't want to do any homework that was reading. And when we did make her read, when we asked her questions about it, she would just say, 'I don't know'. It turned out that she really didn't know. So when we said, 'Take a guess', her guesses were usually wrong. Her teachers had been saying she wasn't concentrating, but actually she wasn't understanding a lot of what she was reading. So we took Noël's advice and we started reading to her. She loved science fiction so we read her some of the science fiction classics because they really held her attention. Of course, she said she didn't want us to read to her and that she wasn't a baby, but we said we would do it for a whole term and then we would see if it made any difference. And it took much less than a term. Pretty soon she was saying she loved reading, and she wasn't making a fuss about her homework any more. Her marks went way up. I think what made it all happen is that she loved the special attention. We also asked her questions every couple of sentences so she had to pay attention. And they were mostly interpretation questions, so she really had to think about the answers.*
>
> Mother of one child, aged 18

Reading comprehension is not really about reading at all! As I explained in Chapter 14, we cannot expect a child to understand something she is reading about if she is not able to understand the same idea when she hears someone talking about it. Reading comprehension starts with listening comprehension.

The skills we need to focus on for improving reading comprehension are:

- Listening comprehension
- Building a store of words that the child has read correctly so many times that these have now become 'sight words', recognisable at a glance without having to be decoded — this frees the child's mind to focus on the meaning of what she is reading
- Accurate and fluent decoding of unfamiliar words

I started to address listening comprehension in Chapter 14, and then in Chapter 15 I explored ways to help children improve their decoding skills and enlarge their store of sight words. In this chapter, I will focus on more advanced listening skills, which can rapidly improve reading comprehension.

Read to your child

Reading to our children is the most effective, as well as the easiest, quickest and most enjoyable, way to improve reading comprehension.

Unless your child is a very skilled and confident reader, the books she is likely to choose to read for her own pleasure usually will not be particularly challenging. They will probably be within the comfort zone of words she can read without a struggle.

But when we read to a child, we can choose more challenging material. Your child will understand the meanings of many words when she hears them in the context of the story, even though she might well have difficulty reading them on her own.

Similarly, children can understand much more complex sentence construction when they are being read to because their brain is engaged in only one task, namely, making mental pictures of what they are hearing. But when children are reading more challenging material, a good part of their working memory must be occupied with the task of decoding, leaving less room for thinking about the ideas and making connections.

So continue the cosy, delightful ritual of reading to your child, even after he has become a good reader. Here are some important guidelines that will make the experience enjoyable and rewarding for both of you and that will result in much improved comprehension. Some of the following guidelines may seem obvious, but others may be new to you:

- As with all habits we want to establish, short daily reading aloud sessions are far more effective than longer but less frequent ones.
- Do not limit reading aloud to your children to the usual time slot just before bedtime. During or right after dinner is another good time because you already have a captive audience. Always have a book or two in your handbag or in the car so that you can read aloud while you are waiting around for an after-school activity to begin. Keep a basket of books in a prominent spot, such as on the coffee table or near the television. If one child is ready to leave the house before the others are, reward him with five or ten minutes of reading aloud. And, of course, Special Time is a perfect opportunity for reading aloud.
- Make sure that your child is physically comfortable. Otherwise he will feel restless and his attention may

wander. He may even complain that the book is 'boring'.

- To maximise your child's concentration, make sure that nothing else is competing for his attention. In particular, he should not be able to hear any screens on in the background as that would be highly distracting for him.
- Start by exploring with your child the front and back cover of the book. Show your child all the interesting information about the book that he can glean from this, even before you start reading. This will help your child to become familiar with authors and illustrators. Read the blurb and together talk about what you can predict from it. Also, talk about what you each may already know about the story.
- If the book contains drawings or photographs, flick through the book and examine them together, seeing what information you can both extract. This usually whets a child's appetite for the book.

Reducing resistance to being read to

Sometimes a child seems uninterested in being read to, or possibly even resistant. Here are some do's and don'ts that can rapidly transform this situation:

- <u>Don't</u> lecture, nag, cajole, bribe, threaten, etc.
- <u>Don't</u> assume that your child is too immature to sit still, listen, absorb and enjoy books the way other children his age can.
- <u>Don't</u> give up.
- <u>Do</u> Prepare for Success with *think-throughs* at a neutral time, several times a day, by asking (not telling) him all about the reading activity:

Who will be reading?

Who will be listening?

Where will you be sitting?

Who will be holding the book?

- <u>Do</u> set a timer for five minutes to begin with, to reassure your child that he will not have to sit still for a very long time.
- <u>Do</u> say that when the timer goes *ding*, you will talk with him about anything else, but for now you're talking only about the book.
- <u>Don't</u> say, *'No, don't, stop'*, when he misbehaves. The immature, impulsive child has heard these words far too many times in his young life, and he may no longer even bother to try and comply. In fact, he may drift into revenge mode, going out of his way to get negative attention.
- <u>Don't</u> wait until your child behaves really well to praise him. That day may never arrive! Instead, be willing to Descriptively Praise tiny improvements, even if he has not yet reached an acceptable standard of behaviour. And remember that phrases such as 'Good boy', 'Well done', and even 'Good listening', do not give the child much useful information.
- <u>Do</u> simplify the text to make it more understandable and more interesting for your child. You can do this by:

    - Substituting more familiar vocabulary
    - Breaking a long, complex sentence into several shorter sentences
    - Adding explanations
    - Leaving out, or briefly summarising, whole paragraphs
    - Repeating key sentences

- <u>Do</u> put lots of expression into your voice. An easy way to do this is to emphasise at least one word in every sentence.
- <u>Do</u> Descriptively Praise any bit of what your child says that is accurate or interesting or imaginative.
- <u>Do</u> point to the appropriate part of the picture as you read the relevant words.
- <u>Do</u> talk <u>a lot</u> about the pictures.
- <u>Do</u> use *trailing statements* (see Chapter 11) to help a child become more confident about answering questions, such as, 'The hunter is carrying . . . (pause for a few seconds to see if he answers; if he doesn't, <u>you</u> finish the sentence) . . . a bow and a quiver full of arrows.' By the time you have said this two or three times, your child will be trying to finish the sentence correctly. You can then respond with a smile and Descriptive Praise.
- <u>Do</u> ask easy questions at first so that your child experiences the satisfaction that comes from understanding a question, answering it correctly, hearing your Descriptive Praise and seeing your pleased smile.
- <u>Do</u> ask the same questions each time you read that book. Soon your child will be anticipating and answering the questions with obvious enjoyment.
- <u>Don't</u> ask any questions of a child who is not paying attention.
- <u>Do</u> read the same story the next time, and start from the beginning all over again. Routines reduce resistance. Familiarity breeds acceptance and then eventually enjoyment.
- <u>Don't</u> have torn or drawn-on books around as that sets a negative example.
- <u>Do</u> sound enthusiastic and excited whenever you are talking about books.

How asking questions improves reading comprehension

Studies have shown that when it comes to being read to, the greatest improvement in comprehension does not come from children simply listening, although that certainly can fire their imagination. What improves reading comprehension the most effectively is asking children questions that require them to think, in particular to deduce, to predict and to consider cause and effect and motive.

Guide your children to answer your questions in complete sentences. This activates the child's brain in unexpected ways and confers several important benefits. Your child will be using more mature thought processes. He will be practising more mature sentence construction and more mature vocabulary. More of what he is listening to will enter his long-term memory. Having to answer in full sentences will help him to listen more carefully. He will soon become proud of being able to speak more maturely and he will realise that he is learning as well as enjoying the experience of being read to.

You will notice in the following examples that most of the questions start with *wh* words: *who, what, when, where, why, how, which*. These *wh* questions require more carefully thought out answers than questions that can be answered with a simple yes or no, such as, 'Did Dorothy ever get back to Kansas?' or, 'Was Huckleberry Finn an orphan?'

Asking memory questions

This is the easiest level of comprehension questions to answer. Memory questions simply ask your child to recall the facts of what she has heard or what she has read:

Who is Harry Potter?

What is Narnia?

In your own words, tell how the slaves escaped to Canada.

Asking interpretation questions

At this more advanced level, your child has to think about the story, not just remember bits of it. He has to make connections:

Tell me what you think about Cinderella's fairy godmother.

What caused the Borrowers to leave their home?

Explain why The Hunger Games is a controversial book.

We must remember that children and teenagers who 'don't like to read' or who 'don't read much' are not simply children who don't want to read. Usually they have experienced that they are not good at reading and they believe that reading will never hold much pleasure for them. As you use the strategies I recommend in this book, your child will become a more skilled reader, and he will naturally start to enjoy reading more. Soon he will define himself as a reader, as someone who loves to read. This is what we are aiming for!

CHAPTER 17

IMPROVING WRITING SKILLS: SENTENCES, PARAGRAPHS, STORIES AND ESSAYS

I've been using the Calmer, Easier, Happier Homework strategies for two years. When my daughter, who's now six, started in Reception, she was one of the youngest, and she made such a fuss about writing her daily journal, saying it was boring, it was too hard and she couldn't think what to write. It seemed like she was just winding me up until I realised she needed Special Time alone with me. I decided to tackle the writing homework in a lot of different ways all at once. I made sure she had a really healthy snack and some exercise in the garden before homework. I did think-throughs asking her what she was going to write. In Reception she only had to write one sentence, but that was like pulling teeth until I learned about the think-throughs and Reflective Listening. Then last year in Year One, she had to write longer stories so I did the spoken word mini-essays that Noël recommends. And now she's in Year Two, and she doesn't mind writing at all. The teacher says she's one of the best. Now I'm using those think-throughs with my middle child, who's in Reception. And the Descriptive Praise really helps all my children to feel proud of themselves.

Mother of three children, aged 6, 4 and 1

Writing is the main way that pupils demonstrate to teachers that they have understood what they have learned and that they remember what they have learned. So just as we want children to learn to express themselves in speech clearly, we also want them to communicate clearly in writing. Writing can also be a form of creative expression. And writing improves children's reading, spelling and punctuation — it even improves their thinking skills.

There are three stages to helping children improve their writing skills. The first is guiding them to overcome any reluctance they may have to writing. Only after a child is cooperative is it possible to teach him the <u>skills</u> needed for writing well. And then we need to train him in the <u>habit</u> of writing well. This will result in improved skills and in increased enthusiasm for writing.

Types of writing that pupils are expected to master

Over the course of a child's school career, she will be expected to develop skills in many different types of writing:

- Narrative (story), which can be about a real or imaginary event
- Letter writing
- Paraphrasing
- Summarising
- Descriptive prose
- Pros and cons essay
- Persuasive essay
- Cause and effect essay
- Process essay, such as a science experiment
- Analytical essay (interpretation)
- Exam answers

A generation ago, most of these types of advanced writing were not introduced until secondary school. Nowadays many are included in the primary school curriculum.

First children learn how to write a sentence that makes sense. Then they learn to write several sentences about a topic, and eventually that becomes a paragraph. This is often the basis of an essay-type answer on exams. Finally, students learn how to group together a number of paragraphs to form an essay.

Each piece of writing has three stages:
1 Planning
2 Writing
3 Proofreading and editing

Stage One: Planning

Many children resist planning, feeling that it is unnecessary and that it uses up valuable time. We need to insist that children learn to plan effectively, and we need to insist that they plan all their writing homework because planning always results in better work.

Planning should be done on paper. Once the child has jotted down a plan, his mind is free to concentrate on developing the plot, describing the characters, using varied vocabulary, thinking about spelling and punctuation, etc.

Most exams ask students to spend five minutes planning an essay. Explain to your child that even if he cannot finish writing his whole essay in an exam, he will still earn some points for the essay if his plan shows that what he intended to write is correct.

Stage Two: Writing

After the planning stage comes the writing stage. Here your child is on his own. Any guidance you want to give him during this stage needs instead to be included in Stage One.

Stage Three: Editing and proofreading

The third stage is the editing and the proofreading stage. If we allow children to skip over or skimp on the first or third stages, we are unintentionally giving them the impression that they don't have to do what it takes to write well.

Strategies for helping children overcome the typical writing problems

1 Reluctance and resistance

There are numerous problems that a child may have with writing, but until he is motivated to practise and improve, it is pointless to try and address these other problems. So the first strategies I will talk about address how to reduce reluctance, resistance and outright refusal.

At the root of this reluctance to write is usually an uncomfortable feeling a child has because he expects to be told off. He expects this because it has happened too often at home, at school and possibly even with a tutor. As a result, he may feel ashamed of his handwriting, his spelling or his punctuation. Understandably, this saps his motivation.

The complaint parents hear most from reluctant writers is 'I can't think of anything to write.' This is where you need to remember that homework is intended to be done by the child. Homework is not, unless specifically stated, supposed to be a joint effort between the parent and the child. So do not do his thinking for him. In fact, parents usually find that any suggestions are immediately shot down, usually with moans of 'That's boring', or 'That will take too long', or 'I still don't know what to write'. Instead:

- Start by asking your child what the task consists of. This is sometimes all that it takes for your child to realise that he does know what to write.

- If that does not get him started, the next step is for the parents to show how to plan a story or essay. Write these six words on a blank page: *who, what, where, when, why* and *how*. Make sure to write these words neatly so that you are setting a good example.

- Ask your child to tell you the answers to these question words, and write down (neatly) what he says. Often this step is enough to help the child realise that he knows what to write.

- But if not, ask your child to tell you a complete sentence for each of those six question words and you write down the sentences. In case you are worried that by writing down the sentences you are doing the child's job for him, remember that this is a temporary strategy and will not be necessary for long.

- As your child is dictating the sentences, ask for descriptive words (such as adjectives and adverbs), and insert them in the sentences.

- If your child says something that is not good grammar, you can say, 'That's not how we say it in English', and then model a better way to say it. This way you are avoiding the word 'grammar', which is often a very confusing topic for children, whereas they can understand that some sentences sound right and some don't.

- Write each sentence that your child dictates on a separate small piece of paper. That way after he has dictated the six sentences, he can move the pieces of paper around until the story is in the correct sequence.

- At that point, have your child copy his dictated sentences neatly and correctly.

This may seem like an awful lot of work for one little piece of writing homework. That's because you are teaching the micro-skills of writing. And teaching does take time and effort on the part of the teacher, as well as the student. If you are willing to tackle the 'I can't think of anything to write' complaint in this way, you will see that it won't be long before your child becomes a competent and confident writer. That will make your investment of time and perseverance worth it!

2 Lack of planning

Most children plunge into a piece of writing without planning. Planning seems like a waste of time because they have not been taught how to plan and because they have not practised it enough to see good results.

As adults we know that if we want to do our best at any writing task, we need all three stages: planning, writing and improving. But your child may not actually be trying to do his best; he may just be wanting to get the ordeal over with. So it is not surprising that he doesn't see the point of planning. Our job is to motivate him to want to do his best, then to teach him how to do his best, then to get him into the habit of regularly doing his best.

Depending on your child's age, the planning will be quite basic or more detailed. A basic type of plan is to jot down the six question words and then write something for each one. That works not only for imaginative stories, but also for many factual essays in subjects other than English, such as History, Science, Geography or Religious Education.

Another type of plan is a *mind map* or *topic web*. Many books have been written about mind-mapping because it is such an effective way of capturing and organising aspects of any topic.

With a mind map, you start by writing the main idea in the centre of a blank page, and then you draw lines radiating outwards from that main idea. On each of these lines you write one aspect of the topic. For example, if the main idea in the centre of the page was *mammals*, one of the lines coming out might be *jungle mammals*, another might be *desert mammals*, and another might be *domestic mammals*. And from each of those lines smaller lines would branch out for the sub-categories, such as *how they raise their young* or *food*. Mind maps are so useful because you can see the main categories and sub-categories at a glance.

Another type of plan that is very effective for narratives is to start with a blank piece of paper and have your child write key words and phrases at random on the paper as they occur to her. Once she has emptied her mind onto the page, she then joins them up on the page in a sensible order.

It is also important to plan the introduction and the conclusion.

As children get older, they will be expected to research topics, and in order to plan they will need to be clear exactly what the topic is. If they are allowed to choose their own topic, children will often choose something far too broad, so you may need to help them narrow it down to something more manageable.

3 Limited or immature vocabulary

Many children use the same words again and again, such as *nice, good* or *bad*. These words do not convey what the child is actually thinking or visualising. Similarly, many children start each sentence in their story or essay with *and then*. Or they may start each sentence with the same noun, rather than switching to a pronoun.

One reason for a limited vocabulary may be poor visualising skills. Or a child may have a good imagination when he is making up a story in his head, but he may not know how to visualise when he is told to. One result of this is stories that give the bare facts but with no elaboration, no interesting details.

To guide children into the habit of starting sentences in more interesting ways, we can make a rule that each sentence has to start with a different word, such as *suddenly, soon, however, often, rarely* or *luckily.*

We can also help children to use words that convey more accurate meanings:

- One way to do this is to challenge ourselves to use more precise language when we are speaking, not only to our children, but also within their hearing. Doing this will inevitably slow us down, which may feel irritating. But parents who have undertaken this challenge report that choosing their words carefully achieves two objectives. Not only does it model more interesting language, but it also helps us to be more positive because we are not being so impulsive.
- We can teach children how to use a thesaurus, which will give them access to many subtle nuances for any word. The old-fashioned type of thesaurus is organised in a way that children may find tricky to master. But many modern ones have a simpler structure, similar to a dictionary, so use those at first. When you are teaching your child how to find the words he wants, start by using a thesaurus designed for younger children. This will be much less daunting.

Descriptions

This game helps expand the child's vocabulary so that he can convey more precise shades of meaning.

In this activity you and your child look carefully at an object, either in real life, in your imaginations or in a picture. Together, take turns coming up with as many adjectives as possible to describe that object. For example, for a flower, you and your child might think of *yellow, white, leafy, soft, light, pretty, small, delicate, sweet-smelling, fluffy, shiny, wet, poisonous*, etc.

Spoken word mini-essays

Help children become comfortable with generating ideas and composing sentences by practising *spoken word mini-essays*. To make it more like a game and to model how to do it, the parent and child should alternate turns (with the parent always being willing to go first if the child is at all reluctant or resistant).

Each of you chooses a topic that you are familiar with and then says five to ten sentences about this topic, starting with an introductory sentence that sets the scene and ending with a conclusion that summarises the mini-essay. As always, find a lot to Descriptively Praise.

As your child gradually becomes more skilled, you can require more sentences, more diverse topics, more mature development of ideas, more precise vocabulary and more interesting sentence construction.

In addition to improving spoken language, this exercise enables your child to practise many important aspects of writing without the slog of having to control his pencil and without the worrying distractions of spelling and punctuation. Therefore each spoken word mini-essay is composed quickly and quite easily. This activity results in rapid, solid improvements in clear communication and confidence. Soon your child or teen will be tackling writing homework with more skill and less resistance.

Synonyms

Another way to help children expand their vocabulary is to make lists of synonyms and near-synonyms. For example, you might say the word *house* and you and your child would come up with types of houses, such as *mansion, bungalow, hut, cottage, castle, shack,* etc. You can do this with verbs as well (eg *walk, saunter, amble*) or adjectives (*large, big, tall, high, huge, enormous, gigantic*) or adverbs (*furiously, crossly, angrily*).

Improving a child's register

Register is about suiting the vocabulary and sentence construction to the task. The concept of using a 'formal' register may seem alien to a child, so it helps to explain that most homework requires writing that 'sounds like a book'. A child may, unless taught otherwise, use an informal, colloquial register in writing. For example, children often write *mum* or *telly*, which is conversational, when they should be writing *mother* or *television*. Older children are less likely to make this mistake, but they will often use clichés because they have heard them spoken and do not realise they are clichés. It seems natural to children to write the way they speak. We need to teach them to avoid clichés, slang and jargon in their writing.

You can turn learning this skill into an enjoyable game by taking turns saying ordinary sentences in colloquial language or slang and challenging each other to rephrase the sentences in more formal language and vice versa.

4 Problems with sequencing

In his writing, the child may put events in the wrong order, or he may leave some important things out altogether. This can make his written work difficult to understand. The following activity teaches the importance of sequencing things in the right order and teaches the child how.

Sequencing steps

(a) Ask your child to explain to you how to do something that he knows how to do very well. It could be making a paper aeroplane, making scrambled eggs, making a bed, washing his hair, cleaning his teeth, building a Lego rocket or walking to school.

(b) As he tells you how he would do it, write each of his sentences on a separate small piece of paper.

(c) Lay the pieces of paper on the table, leaving gaps wherever the child has left out some important information.

(d) Ask leading questions to guide him to discover what steps in the process would be needed to fill the gaps.

(e) Write the missing steps on separate pieces of paper, and have your child put them in the right order on the table.

(f) Once all of the steps are written, mix up the pieces of paper, and have your child put them in the correct order again.

Sequencing stories

Here is another game that helps children to become more skilled at sequencing.

You and your child think of a familiar story, one that you both know well. Together you tell this story, each of you adding the next sentence. When it is your turn to add a sentence, add description or more detail rather than moving the action forward. When it is your child's turn to add the next sentence, he is likely to move the action forward because children are usually more interested in action than in description. If your child leaves out an important part of the story or muddles the order, correct him by asking questions, and then continue the story. Not only does this game reinforce sequencing skills, but it also models how to enrich a story by adding description and detail.

5 Lack of shared background knowledge

A child's writing may be difficult to understand because he is assuming that the reader knows something that the child has not actually included in the story or essay. To write clearly, the writer needs to know what background information will be known to the reader. You can guide your child to become more aware of this *shared background knowledge* by asking him, in daily conversation, to clarify anything he says that is not immediately clear. For example, if your child says, 'Mr. Smith said my report was really good', you can say, 'I know your teacher's name is Miss Jones, so I'm guessing Mr. Smith might be a helper?'

6 Not enough description

When a child concentrates on the action in a story and leaves out description, the result is boring. Make a rule that for narratives, whether imaginary or factual, each sentence of action must be followed by two sentences of description. This can be description of the action or of the effect of the action. The child can describe the motives of the person who did something or can describe the surroundings.

To help a child come up with descriptions, have her imagine the scene as if she is in a darkened cinema, looking at a screen. Ask her to tell you what she can picture on the screen. Start your questions with *who, what, when, where, why, how,* and *which*:

What colour is the boat?

How big is the dog?

Where is the treasure chest?

These questions will help your child sharpen her visualising skills.

7 Sentences that are too short

Some children, boys in particular, write sentences that are very short and that consequently sound choppy and awkward. This is because boys tend to speak in shorter sentences, whereas girls, even from an early age, tend to use more complex sentences, which include more clauses.

Combining sentences

The following activity improves sentence construction, resulting in more complex and more mature sentences.

Write two short sentences, such as, 'I have a dog. My dog is big'. Show your child how to combine them into one sentence, which in this case would be 'I have a big dog'. When he has mastered that basic stage of combining two sentences, you can move on to more complicated sentences, where three or more elements are combined, including adjectives and adverbs.

8 Incorrect sentence construction (often known as 'bad grammar')

Children need to learn to speak correctly before they are likely to write correctly. So let's start by setting a good example, practising speaking correctly when our children are around. Their speech will be influenced by our speech. We can also Descriptively Praise our children whenever they speak maturely.

When a child makes a mistake in a spoken sentence, model the correct sentence, and then have her repeat the sentence correctly.

9 Not proofreading carefully

One of the biggest writing problems is that children assume that the task is complete as soon as they have finished writing. As adults we know that to do one's best requires checking and often rechecking. It is the rare child or teen who is keen to do this or who even knows how to do it well. Proofreading and editing one's written work is such an important skill and habit to establish that I devote a separate chapter to it: Chapter 20.

10 Handwriting problems

Some children find the physical act of writing very difficult, sometimes even painful. Naturally they try to write as little as possible. In Chapter 19, I give suggestions for how to improve handwriting and how to make writing physically more comfortable.

CHAPTER 18

IMPROVING SPELLING AND PUNCTUATION

> *My little girl has always been a good speller, but my older boy used to be terrible at spelling. It used to annoy me that he wouldn't even try. Part of the problem was that when I would practise spelling with him, his younger sister would answer because she knew how to spell his spelling words. I could see he felt terrible about that. My wife and I realised that getting angry with him wasn't working so we decided on a much more positive approach. We taught him the spelling words in word families, and we did lots of cumulative review so that he didn't forget the spelling words from earlier in the term. We also needed to do lots of Reflective Listening at first. And when we had our Special Time, if it was my turn to choose what to do I would bring out word games like Boggle and Upwords. Upwords actually got him into looking words up in the dictionary. He got a lot of Descriptive Praise for that. He's very competitive and he wanted to win, and actually he's very good now — good at Upwords and good at spelling. And it's not just spelling. Now he takes his time over his homework and he's very proud of doing good work. I never thought I'd see the day.*
>
> Father of two children, aged 10 and 7

For many centuries the spelling of words in the English language was a completely personal matter. There were no rules about how words should be spelled so people could spell words however they wanted. Shakespeare famously spelled his own surname many different ways.

At a certain point in history, spelling was regularised, and it became the mark of an educated person to use what was from then on considered to be correct spelling. Nowadays people are still often judged on their spelling. Someone who spells well is considered to be not only better educated, but also more intelligent and more sensible. We can see the fallacy in this, but the perception persists. Children who do not think of themselves as good spellers often feel ashamed, although they may hide it by making fun of their poor spelling. This uncomfortable feeling can colour their whole school experience because spelling is an aspect of all written work, regardless of the subject. Being able to spell well contributes to a child's self-respect. We may wish this were not true, but sadly it is.

Poor spelling is marked down in exams. And when young people enter the world of work, it has been shown that even one spelling mistake on a CV can result in that CV ending up in the bin. A number of studies have shown that office workers with poor spelling do not get promoted as often as those with good spelling and that blue-collar workers with poor spelling rarely make the leap to office work.

Why some children are naturally good spellers and others are not

Children who are good spellers usually do not have to think much about how to spell because they tend to have a good visual-symbolic memory. They often read a lot and this results in correct spellings being imprinted on their brain many thousands of times. Good spellers tend to be interested in words. And good spellers often pride themselves on being good spellers so they are more likely to check their work carefully before they hand it in. Therefore good spellers tend to become even better spellers.

Children of any age who are not good spellers can improve their ability to spell accurately. They may never become excellent spellers, but they can become adequate spellers. They can learn strategies to improve their spelling and to catch the spelling mistakes that they do make.

When children who are poor spellers are writing an unfamiliar word, they do not automatically focus on the link between the sound of the word and what letters they are going to write. Sometimes this is due purely to impulsivity. But it can also be due to a genetically inherited difficulty with what is called 'phoneme awareness', which means awareness of the sounds that make up words. If this difficulty is significant it is considered to be an aspect of a specific learning difficulty, such as dyslexia. Without targeted, effective intervention, poor spellers often become even worse spellers.

Some children are poor spellers simply because they have never been taught the spelling rules and patterns that govern spelling in our language. This, however, is rare. It is much more common that a child <u>has</u> been taught these facts, but in a way that did not engage his interest. So he was not really paying attention during those lessons and consequently did not absorb this important information.

It is understandable that a child who finds spelling difficult will naturally want to avoid thinking about it. She may feel embarrassed about her spelling mistakes, especially if she has been corrected a lot by teachers and parents. If a younger sibling spells better, this compounds the shame. The result is that a poor speller does not improve over time, unless effective interventions are put into place.

Realistic spelling goals

No one is expected to be able to spell all the words in the English language correctly. Generally children are expected to be able to consistently spell correctly the words they encounter in their school reading and the words they are likely to use in their school writing. They are expected to be able to take a sensible guess at spelling unfamiliar words by remembering the rules and patterns they have been taught and by keeping in mind the most common spelling mistakes.

The guidelines below explain which words children should be able to spell correctly at which ages. This is of course only approximate because different schools, and indeed individual teachers within a school, will have their own standards for what is acceptable:

- By c. 6 years old: phonetically regular words, eg *clap, blink, crop*
- By c. 8 years old:
  a) words with consistent patterns, eg *train, bridge, clear*
  b) high-frequency words that are phonetically irregular, eg *listen, their, many*
- By c. 9 years old:
  a) words from their own life
     family members
     addresses of home and school
     friends
     teachers
     school subjects
  b) general knowledge
     months of the year
     days of the week
     holidays
     countries and cities
- By c. 10 years old: specialised terminology of science, history, etc.
- At every age: words on the weekly spelling lists

How to overcome your child's resistance to thinking about spelling

We can do this within the context of homework, but we also need to do it out of context, at times other than during home-work. Shortly I will explain some strategies for improving spelling during homework. Here I want to talk about how we can help overcome children's resistance at other times of day:

1   Devote five minutes a day, six days a week to spelling prac-tice. Set a timer, and put it out of reach so your child cannot fiddle with it. Be sure to stop the spelling practice as soon as the timer goes *ding* even if that is mid-word. This will reas-sure your child that when you say five minutes of spelling practice, it really is only five minutes. Even a child who dreads spelling soon realises that he can cope with five minutes of it.

2   To build a solid foundation and to boost confidence, start with the easiest words. If necessary, start by having your child practise spelling phonetically regular one-syllable words. If your child does not yet reliably know how to spell all the vowel sounds, have him practise spelling words that all have the same vowel sound, eg *cat, bag, snap, fan, rag.* Include non-words, eg *rab, lan, vap, tas.*

3   Teach word families together. For example, you can teach *hope, hoped, hoping, hopeless, hopeful and hopefully* at the same time. Because we learn by association, these words will all go into your child's memory in a group, thus reduc-ing the processing load.

4   Poor spellers often have poor handwriting. When they are practising spelling by writing out the words, they are not able to just focus on how to spell because they also have to pay attention to controlling their pen or pencil in order to keep their letters on the line, keep their letters the right size and

form their letters properly so they are the right shape. So rather than having children practise spelling by writing out the words, have them spell the words by arranging letter tiles in the right order. Not only is this probably more fun for your child, but his spelling will improve more rapidly because he is focusing only on the spelling. Letter tiles can be bought or made out of card. Make sure that the letters on the tiles are lower-case.

5 Capture and display your child's successes. Once she has spelled several words correctly using the letter tiles, with your mobile phone take a photograph of the words laid out on the table, and make a big point of showing this to another adult — either your partner or another family member or maybe even your child's teacher.

6 Remember to Descriptively Praise even small successes:

You remembered the silent e so this word says cape, not cap.

You weren't sure how to make the e sound in bread. You remembered there was another vowel so you put one in.

7 Even though this spelling practice lasts only five minutes, and even though you are doing your best to make it enjoyable and rewarding, it is quite possible that a child who thinks of himself as a poor speller will dread it and resist it at first. Remember to do lots of Reflective Listening:

It looks like thinking about spelling feels awful.

Maybe you're worried you'll get them wrong?

8 There are many amusing poems that highlight the inconsistencies of English spelling. These can be used to teach spelling. Similarly, there are funny sentences that entertain

and teach spelling at the same time. You can find these on the internet.

9 Never say that you are not good at spelling or even that as a child you were not good at spelling. Parents often say this sort of thing to empathise with their child; unfortunately it often has the unintended result of making the child think that spelling is not really very important. You can certainly say that as a child you struggled with spelling, but that you overcame the problem, if that is true. This will set your child a good example. It will show him that he does not need to be a poor speller forever.

Strategies for helping children to become interested in spelling

It may feel as if your child is so resistant to even thinking about spelling that you couldn't possibly imagine him ever being interested in words or curious about how words are spelled. From my long experience working with children and teens, I know that this state of affairs is reversible. At any age our children are influenced by our attitudes, our words and our actions.

With the letter tiles that I have mentioned, you can have your child spell out his name or other family members' names and then rearrange the letters to make other words.

One very effective way to awaken a child's interest in spelling is to play word games. You may like this idea, but you may be worried that your child would make a fuss or possibly even refuse to play these games with you. Yes, your child may make a fuss at first, especially if you spring it on him unexpectedly. That is why *think-throughs*, which I explained in Chapter 6, are so useful.

One result of children and teens spending too much time in front of a screen is that they become much less interested in other leisure activities, including word games. You may not know how to wean him off this screen dependence. In the companion volume, *Calmer, Easier, Happier Parenting*, I explain how you can get back in charge of the electronics in your home. One benefit of significantly reducing screen time is that suddenly there is more time available to play games as a family. Children (and even teenagers) will gradually become more enthusiastic about non-screen activities.

Routines reduce resistance so it is a good idea to have a set time, a couple of times a week, when you and your child will play word games together. Some are what are known as box and board games, some are paper and pencil games, and some require no equipment whatsoever.

Some of the box and board games that are very useful for teaching children about spelling and helping them to become interested in spelling are Boggle, Junior Scrabble and Upwords. If your child is not yet confident, you can eliminate or reduce the competitive element so that he does not feel like a failure. You can take away the anxiety of having a time limit by not using a timer. You can play as a team, rather than against each other. A way to introduce a bit of competition, without making a child anxious, is to play together and add up everyone's combined scores. Then play again and together try and beat your earlier joint score.

Paper and pencil spelling games

Find the little words

Have your child choose a long word, and together make smaller words from those letters. For example, if the long word was *conversation*, your child could make *sat, vat, tin, nit, rat, not, rot, cot,* etc.

Write as many

You and your child can decide what you will write as many of. It could be two-letter words or three-letter words; it could be words that begin with or end with or include a certain letter or combination of letters. It could be a category such as animals, colours, occupations, books, famous people from history, etc. This game can be timed or untimed. Points are scored for correct spelling of correct answers.

Flowerman

This next game is similar to Hangman, but less gruesome! Make a flower by adding the stem, leaves and petals each time the child guesses a letter that is not in the word. As you add a piece of the flower, explain whether the letter that your child guessed was a reasonable or an unreasonable guess.

Spelling games that require no equipment

I Spy

We are all familiar with the game I Spy. You can make it easier or more challenging by using the first two or three letters of the object, by using the last letter or by giving a clue, etc.

Ghost

In the game Ghost, the first person thinks of a word and says the first letter, without saying what word she is thinking of. The next person in the circle thinks of a word that starts with that letter and says the second letter in the word they are thinking of. They may, of course, be thinking of a completely different word. The third person has to think of a word start-ing with the first two letters already spoken. The aim of the game is to avoid saying the last letter in a word. Each time that happens, the person who completed the word becomes a G, then an H, then an O, etc.

For children whose spelling skills are not yet good enough for Ghost, here is an easier variation. One person chooses a word, announces what the word is and says the first letter aloud. The next person says the next letter in that word. You can correct spelling mistakes as the game progresses. You can explain whether the next letter a child suggests is a reasonable or an unreasonable guess.

Helping children understand why a word is spelled the way it is

Many people assume that the way to improve spelling is through memorising. It is true that some syllables in some words defy reason and need to be memorised, but most sylla-bles in English do follow a rule or pattern. But poor spellers often do not know what the pattern is; they may not even real-ise that these patterns exist. We would like to think that schools teach this effectively. Sadly, many schools teach spell-ing too quickly, too sketchily or in a dry, uninteresting way. Sometimes a child switches off because he is already convinced that he is no good at spelling.

Therefore it falls to the parents to teach, or reteach, spelling rules and patterns. It is not enough for us to explain these rules and patterns. The child needs to be able to explain clearly what the rules and patterns are, and she needs to demonstrate this knowledge by spelling words correctly using the letter tiles.

A number of frequently misspelled words are compound words, which means that they are made up of two smaller words. Compound words instantly become easier to spell once we show a child the smaller words within the larger word. For example, the word *maybe* is often misspelled, with the *y* missing. Once children understand that *maybe* is a combination of *may* and *be*, they are much more likely to remember to write the *y*. Similarly, the word *tomorrow* is often misspelled with *mm* because children have a vague sense that there are some double letters in that word, but they are not sure which letters to double. Once children know that *tomorrow* is made up of two words, *to* and *morrow* (which is an old-fashioned word for *morning*), they no longer spell it with *mm*.

Children are often interested in the differences in spelling between the United States and the United Kingdom. You can find examples of these differences in books and on the internet.

For poor spellers, an annoying characteristic of the English language is that many words include an unaccented syllable where it is not possible to hear what the vowel is, for example the second syllable in *doctor*. This sound is called a 'schwa'. We can teach children to find a longer word in the same word family. In the longer word the likelihood is that the unaccented syllable will now be accented, enabling us to hear what the vowel is. For example, we cannot hear what the vowel should be in the final syllable of *regular*. But when we think of *regularity*, we can hear that the vowel in question is an *a*.

Principles of memorising spelling

One principle of memorising that is often overlooked is that it is easier to memorise something that we understand. This is so obvious that it seems we hardly need to say it. But children are often expected to learn to spell words whose meaning they are not quite clear about. So first we have to make sure they understand the meanings of the words they have to learn and can use them correctly in sentences.

In Chapter 11 I outlined the most effective strategies for memorising. For example, *attempting to retrieve* information signals the brain that this information is important and needs to be stored in the long-term memory. The *attempts to retrieve* need to happen at *lengthening intervals*. This trains the brain to store the information for longer and longer periods of time. And I talked about *cumulative review*. We cannot expect children to remember the spelling of words that they studied briefly a few weeks ago. We need to make sure that they revise those spellings over many weeks.

A mistake that some teachers and spelling workbooks make is to group together words that sound alike but do not follow a consistent spelling pattern, such as *bear, hair, care*. This confuses children. For most of us, the strongest processing channel is the visual, so we need to group together words that look similar, such as *bear, hear, head*. What is similar about these words is the *ea*, even though the *ea* makes a different sound in each of the words.

Using spelling mnemonics

Mnemonics use the power of association to reduce the memorising load on the brain. Here are a few common spelling mnemonics that children often find very useful:

- The word *friend* is often misspelled, but if you teach children to say, 'I am a friend to the end,' they soon remember that the word *friend* ends with *end*.

- Children can remember that all the vowels in the word *cemetery* are *e* if you say something like 'Some people would find a cemetery scary, and they might scream; they might say e, e, e.'
- Many people have trouble spelling *practise* and *practice*. Think of *advise* and advice. We know that *advise* is the verb and *advice* is the noun because we can easily hear the difference in that pair of words. We cannot hear the difference between *practise* and *practice*, but by referring back to *advise* and *advice* we can remember that *practice* with a *c* is the noun and *practise* with an *s* is the verb.
- Your child can remember how to spell *piece* if she thinks of a *piece of pie*. The first part of *piece* is *pie*.

Teaching dictionary skills

When a child misspells a word or wants to know the meaning of a word, it is very tempting to say, 'Look it up in the dictionary.' This turns children off dictionaries because they often find the process difficult, time-consuming and discouraging.

To take the mystery and fear out of dictionaries, sit down with your child once a week or so and together browse through the dictionary just for fun, not at a time when she needs to look up the spelling or meaning of a word for homework. She will become familiar with a dictionary, and you will be able to explain many aspects that she probably finds confusing.

You may need to teach your child how to use a dictionary accurately and quickly. This is often taught quite sketchily in school. You may even need to show how to open the dictionary to approximately the right place. Without this skill, children may open the dictionary at random, or they may start at the very beginning when they are looking for a word that starts with *p*. Teach your child that the letters *a* through to *j* are towards the beginning of the alphabet and the letters *r* through to *z* are towards the end.

Once your child has located the correct initial letter, you will probably need to explain what the words at the top of the page are for.

In theory, children learn how to put words in alphabetical order at school, and they generally master alphabetising by the first letter. But when faced with having to put in alphabetical order a number of words that all have the same first letter, children often get confused. You may need to have them practise this until they become skilled.

Even once they have located the word they are looking for, many children are still confused because the definitions are often not very user-friendly. Therefore I recommend that at first even teenagers be given dictionaries for children, rather than adult dictionaries.

There is a type of dictionary called a spelling dictionary that does not include definitions, except to differentiate between words that sound the same but are spelled differently. These are very useful.

Use an exercise book to make a dictionary of the words that your child has difficulty spelling or is likely to need to know how to spell. She will be able to refer to this again and again, and it will help her to become self-reliant.

Set a good example by keeping a dictionary handy, eg near the dinner table. Make a point, in front of your children, of looking up the spellings or the meanings of words. Your enthusiasm will start to make dictionaries interesting for children.

Strategies for improving spelling during homework

In Chapter 5, I recommended that all homework be divided into three stages. Stage One is the *think-through*, Stage Two is when your child does the work without any help, and Stage Three is the improving stage. Here is how to handle spelling at each of these stages.

Stage One: The think-through

In Stage One, make sure that your child has handy his home-made dictionary of words he often misspells. In addition, ask your child what words he might need for the homework he is about to do. You can list these words for him to ensure the correct spelling. This list will also function as an aide-memoire for the content of what he is going to write in Stage Two. It will help him remember his ideas, and the order of the words you have listed will show him the order of what he is planning to write.

Stage Two: Your child works on his own

In Stage Two, as your child is writing, he may ask you how to spell a word. Don't tell him! I am aware that this advice is contrary to what parents are usually told. Make sure during the Stage One *think-through* to clarify that in Stage Two your child will be on his own. He will have to consult the dictionary you have provided for him or his little home-made dictionary or the list of words you have written down for him, or he will have to take a sensible guess. During Stage Two, don't give a hint or a clue or a prompt. Don't even say whether the word is spelled correctly or incorrectly. Remember that in Stage Two the child is working on his own. This will foster self-reliance and more mature problem-solving skills.

Stage Three: The improving stage

In Stage Three you can address spelling by underlining or listing the words your child has spelled <u>correctly</u>. This is the opposite of what we generally do. Usually we notice and point out the misspelled words, which is very demotivating, especially for a child who already thinks of himself as a poor speller.

As you list the correctly spelled words, your child will be watching you with interest. He will notice which words you are not writing down, and he is likely to try and fix the spelling of those. When he has corrected a spelling, you can add that word to your list of correctly spelled words.

For the words that are still misspelled, here is a way to help children start to learn the spellings. On a blank piece of paper, write all the words he misspelled, but write them correctly, and do not write them in the order that they appear in the child's written work. Your child looks at the list of correct spellings and chooses a word. Then he needs to find where in his writing to put this word. This will teach him to pay attention to how words are spelled much more effectively than if he simply rubbed out his misspelling and wrote in your correct spelling.

Give a *diagnostic response* (see Chapter 11) that explains why your child made the mistake he did. For example, if he spelt *bread* as *bred,* you can say, 'Since the *a* is silent, you didn't know that it needed to be in there.' And then follow up with some questions:

So what is the silent letter in bread?

What are the two vowels in bread?

Which vowel comes first?

Which vowel is silent?

How do you spell bread?

Asking those questions takes less than a minute.

What to do when your child asks you how to spell a word outside of Stage Two

In Stage Two of the homework you won't be talking about spelling, or about anything else for that matter. But you will be talking about spelling in Stages One and Three, and your child may also ask you about spelling outside of homework, when he is engaged in spontaneous writing.

- Avoid talking about any words as difficult to spell or hard. Don't use the phrases 'can't spell' or 'don't know how to spell'. Instead, you can say something much more neutral:

    Which part of the word are you wondering about?

    *Are you wondering if there is one **s** or two?*

    You probably know how it ends. Is it the beginning that you're wondering about?

- Tell your child the pattern or the rule that the word he is wanting to spell follows. Then his brain needs to work out how to apply that pattern to the word he is wondering about. For example, if he asks how to spell *swimming*, you could say, 'You need to double the consonant.'
- Ask him to take a sensible guess in writing rather than just spelling the word aloud. This will curb his impulsivity. You can then look at what he has written and give a *diagnostic response*.

Teaching children how to remember the spelling of the words in their weekly spelling list

Most schools give children a list of spelling words to learn each week. The following week, children are given a new list, and the previous weeks' lists are rarely referred to. The problem is that last week's words are not yet embedded in the child's long-term memory. Without *cumulative review* and *attempting to retrieve*, those words will soon evaporate from his short-term memory. This is what makes spelling tests and studying for them a frustrating waste of time for so many children. We need to make sure that the spelling lists from previous weeks are regularly revised using the memorising strategies explained in Chapter 11. And the words need to be learned in sentences, rather than in isolation. Otherwise it is entirely possible for a child to spell a word correctly on the weekly spelling test, but then misspell the same word later the same day in a story or essay.

Children who are not good spellers or who are not confident about their spelling will often copy their spelling words incorrectly from the board because it is not easy for their brain to hold several letters in their mind's eye at the same time. Looking at the whole word just confuses them. The way to overcome this is for the parent to cover everything but the first syllable. Have the child look at the first syllable and then write the first syllable (neatly of course), holding those few letters in his mind. Then do the same thing with the next syllables. Over time, this technique improves the short-term visual memory.

Children who are poor spellers do not easily visualise a word correctly, even if they have just looked at it. We can teach a child or teenager to visualise better by having her close her eyes and imagine that she is in a cinema with a big screen in front of her. First show your child the word to be learned and ask her to put that word up on her big mental screen. Start with one-syllable words while your child is learning how to visualise. Once your child can 'see' the word in her mind, have her read off the letters from her mental screen. As she is imagining herself looking at her screen, ask questions like:

What's the first letter you see?

What's the last letter?

What's the vowel that comes after the s?

What's the next to the last letter?

Questions like this will sharpen your child's ability to keep the word on her mental screen. It may take your child a few days or a few weeks to master the skill of visualising one-syllable words. Next have her visualise two-syllable words, and then three and four, etc. At that point you would be asking questions such as:

What are the letters in the first syllable?

*What are the letters that make the **ver** sound?*

What are the letters in the next-to-last syllable?

Tell me all the letters in all the syllables.

Make sure that your child spells each syllable separately from the next syllable, pausing briefly in between each syllable. This method is highly effective at improving spelling.

How you can use letter tiles to improve spelling

Step 1 From a pool of letter tiles on the table, the child picks out the letters of a particular word by referring to the correct spelling of the word on the weekly spelling list. Looking carefully and matching the tiles to the word on the list starts the process of learning to spell the word.

Step 2 The child then jumbles up the letter tiles and re-arranges them again in the right order to spell the word correctly, referring back to the word list only if necessary. Have your child do this until he is putting the letter tiles in the right order without having to look back at the spelling list.

Step 3 This step teaches the child to visualise the words in his mind. The parent turns one of the letter tiles in the word face down so that the letter is not visible and the child spells the word aloud while looking at the tiles. Obviously, he cannot see the letter on the tile that is turned over so he is visualising that letter. Do this several times, each time turning a different letter tile face down. Once your child can spell the word this way, with one letter hidden, turn two letter tiles at a time face down and have your child spell aloud the letters he sees and the letters he is visualising. Do this several times, varying which letters you hide.

Step 4 Once your child has mastered Step 3, he will usually be able to spell the whole word even when all the letter tiles are turned face down. He is visualising the letter tiles as he spells.

For older children, you can do Steps 1 through to 4 with multi-syllable words by having a syllable on each tile.

Step 5 Once your child can say all the letters or all the syllables, it is time for him to practise writing the words, neatly of course, keeping his letters on the line and making his tall letters tall and his small letters small.

Step 6 Have your child tell you which bit of the word seems tricky. You may be surprised by what you hear. For a phonetically regular word such as *trip,* you may feel that there is nothing tricky, but your child may think the *r* is tricky. Poor spellers often leave out the second letter in a consonant cluster because they don't register the second sound. Or he may point to the *i* because he may not really be absolutely sure which short vowel sounds go with which letters.

Step 7 Have your child colour with a marker or crayon the letters he thinks are tricky.

Step 8 Then he turns the word face down and tells you about the tricky letters.

Step 9 Once he can do this, which may take several times, have him write the whole word from memory.

These ways of teaching spelling are usually far more effective for poor spellers than the often recommended 'look, cover, write, check' method. That is because a poor speller can easily look too briefly, cover, write the word incorrectly and then not even notice it is wrong when he checks. It is much more effective to guide the child to look carefully at the parts of the word.

Punctuation

Many children and teens who are poor spellers also have persistent difficulties, year after year, with punctuation. The root of the problem is usually weak attention to visual detail, often compounded by not really knowing the purposes that the different types of punctuation serve.

As with spelling, punctuation can be taught and improved within the daily homework time. During the Stage One *think-through* ask leading questions, and during Stage Three make a point of noticing and Descriptively Praising correct punctuation.

Outside of homework time, or on days when the homework that has been set does not take up all of the time allotted for it, you can play a game that rapidly improves punctuation. You and your child each write a short paragraph, purposefully making several punctuation errors in each sentence. Children enjoy making mistakes on purpose! Then swap paragraphs and, using a different coloured pen, you each need to find and correct the other person's deliberate mistakes. This usually leads to a lively discussion and to a lot of learning.

CHAPTER 19

IMPROVING HANDWRITING

I used to find my son very puzzling. He was clearly bright. He loved everything to do with science and history, and he was very good at maths, but he hated anything to do with writing. So even in the subjects that he was good at, he would try not to do his homework if it was writing homework. And creative writing was the worst. He complained that his hand hurt, his arm hurt, his back hurt. At first my husband and I didn't believe him. Then we realised there wasn't going to be one simple, quick solution to this. We had to change a lot of things. He's quite small for his age and his feet were dangling, so we got him a chair with a footrest. That helped his posture a lot. We used Blu-Tack to keep his paper in the right position on the table so that he wouldn't twist himself into a weird position. We had him do ten minutes of handwriting practice every day before he started his home-work, as Noël suggests. And he had a terrible pencil grip with his thumb wrapped around his other fingers. It made him press very hard. So when he was doing his handwriting practice he had to use the right pencil grip. We never would have been able to make all these changes if we hadn't known about think-throughs. We did think-throughs every day about handwriting and used lots of Descriptive Praise. And in the first week or two we had to do so much Reflective Listening! The Special Time also really helped because it made him want us to be proud of him — just like Noël said. The neatness of his handwriting improved very quickly. He stopped saying it hurt to write. And he stopped making a fuss about writing homework. Writing will probably never be his favourite thing, but now he's not avoiding it.

Mother of one boy, aged 9

For the first ten years of a child's school career, he is likely to be judged on his handwriting. Many parents and teachers seem to believe that sloppy handwriting is almost a character flaw. For those children whose handwriting is not considered good enough, this can lead to issues with self-esteem. Even though most of what adults write nowadays is typed, legible handwriting is still necessary for children. And many would argue that the self-discipline required to improve one's handwriting is an important habit for children and teens to develop.

Realistic handwriting goals for children and teens

When a parent or teacher is reading what a child has written, it is not enough to be able to guess the word from the context. Each word, taken separately, needs to be legible. To achieve this goal, the following should be happening most of the time:

- Letters sitting on the line
- Letters formed correctly
- Tall letters tall, small letters small
- Upper-case letters used correctly
- Correct spacing between words and between letters within a word
- About eight words to a line on standard-sized paper
- Joined-up writing (usually by age eight).
- Writing is neat, not just where it matters for a good mark, but throughout the child's day

How problems with handwriting affect homework

Children with poor handwriting often feel a great deal of shame about this, even though they may appear to laugh it off. Ironically, feeling bad about their writing leads them to rush through their work to get the unpleasant experience over with so they end up, yet again, doing a poor job of writing.

The child may resist writing, sometimes to the point of crying, tantrums, running away, hiding his homework or even lying. Or he may start each day's homework session in a relatively cheerful mood and gradually become more frustrated and irritable and want to give up before the homework is finished. As a result, he may fall behind in his work, which adds to his stress. For this child, homework often takes far too long. The child loses concentration, may experience real physical pain or discomfort and can become exhausted so that the quality of his work suffers. Plus, he is left with not enough free time to recuperate emotionally.

The child may have to concentrate so much of his attention on forming the letters correctly and keeping them the right size and on the line that there is no room left in his working memory for other aspects of writing, such as the development of ideas, sequencing, spelling and punctuation. This results in what are often considered to be careless mistakes.

A child with poor handwriting usually writes the very minimum that will be acceptable to a parent or teacher. It is often said of this child that he is 'easily satisfied', but that does not describe how the child is feeling at all. He is feeling very *dis*satisfied and is trying to get the writing over with as quickly as possible.

As a result, the content and style of this child's written work is often quite immature and truncated; it does not match the content and style of his speaking, which may be quite mature and articulate.

The causes of handwriting problems

Children with messy handwriting are often thought of as lazy. Parents and teachers may assume that these children simply cannot be bothered to slow down and think about their writing. And watching these children write may reinforce that belief. They often rush through their work and appear to have no concern for doing it well. But what looks like laziness is really part of a vicious circle. Children with messy handwriting start out with a genuine difficulty.

And because they are frequently corrected or told off, they soon get discouraged. All that correcting just reinforces their view of themselves as someone who cannot write well, so they give up trying to improve. They develop the habit of rushing through their work because writing is such an unrewarding experience.

The underlying causes of poor handwriting are usually problems with spatial awareness and fine-motor control, which includes eye-hand coordination. These difficulties may simply be due to immaturity, or they may be actual deficiencies, which are often genetically inherited. Spatial awareness refers to how the brain perceives objects in space, in particular their location and size, sometimes also shape. Improving spatial awareness rapidly improves handwriting. Fine motor control describes how the brain sends messages to, and receives messages from, the small muscles in the body. Gross-motor control, on the other hand, is about how the brain sends messages to, and receives messages from, the large muscles. The large muscles are found in our arms, legs and trunk. The small muscles are found in our hands, feet, neck, face and also our sphincters. It is possible for a child to have average or even excellent gross-motor skills and yet have poor fine-motor skills.

Mature fine motor skills are necessary for many important aspects of schoolwork and homework — not only writing, but also drawing, cutting, gluing, using a ruler, etc. In addition to handwriting problems, children with relatively poor fine motor control are likely to be messy eaters for their age. They may want to eat with their fingers because they find managing cutlery a challenge. They may make a fuss about getting dressed, which may seem like laziness or contrariness, but is often fuelled by genuine difficulty with buttons and zippers and shoelaces. This is often, but not always, a child who does not like to draw and does not enjoy doing puzzles.

If the handwriting problem is severe enough, a child may be diagnosed with dysgraphia. *Dys* means difficulty and *graphia* means writing. Dysgraphia simply describes a significant difficulty with writing in a child of at least average ability who has learned to read. But the term does not tell us anything about the causes of the difficulties.

Dysgraphia is often a characteristic of other special educational needs, especially dyspraxia, ADHD or autism spectrum disorders, sometimes dyslexia. But dysgraphia also exists in children who show no evidence of any other learning difficulties. In those cases, there is often a parent or other close family member who shows signs of dysgraphia as well.

If the dysgraphia is particularly problematic, a child may be diagnosed with dyspraxia, which is a neurological disorder that affects coordination. If the problem is milder, it might be called 'dyspraxic-type symptoms'.

If you suspect that your child is having an unusual degree of difficulty mastering handwriting or other fine motor skills, it is a good idea to take him to be assessed by an occupational therapist, who will be able to pinpoint the causes of the problem and will suggest exercises that can strengthen the weak areas. Parents are often surprised at how quickly handwriting can improve from doing these exercises.

If you realise that these characteristics describe your child, you can choose to do nothing, hoping that he will grow out of this problem. Certainly his fine-motor skills will improve with time, although probably much more slowly than would be expected. And in the meantime he is drifting into bad habits.

Instead, I recommend that parents undertake teaching and training. Fine motor skills <u>can</u> be improved. It requires only a very small amount of daily practice. The key is for the child to be practising micro-skills that are a tiny bit of a stretch for him, but that he is capable of doing with only a bit more concentration than usual.

Realistically, some children are not likely ever to become neat, fluent, fast writers. They will always need to focus so much attention on this one aspect of their work that other more interesting, and more important, aspects get short-changed.

These children and teens may also benefit from being taught keyboard skills early on so that their poor handwriting becomes a non-issue. This is not necessarily a simple solution because children with fine motor skills problems may have difficulty learning to type as well. But usually they find typing easier and more enjoyable than writing by hand. Another option is voice-recognition software that circumvents the problems of poor fine motor skills altogether.

Children and teens with a diagnosed learning difficulty may be able to get extra time in exams or may be able to use a laptop or a scribe. In addition, you can ask the school to recognise that, even with good intentions, your child has to write very slowly to be legible. A way to even the playing field for this child is to accept shorter written work or oral answers.

Improving handwriting

What typically happens before parents know about teaching handwriting through *think-throughs* to improve spatial awareness is that the child produces messy handwriting and gets told off for it. The frustrated parent may then tell the child to redo the work, in the hope that this will teach him to pay attention to writing neatly. This rarely works. It is bound to cause resentments, unless we have made it clear ahead of time that a child will have to redo work if he does not reach a certain standard. And even after the work has been redone, you probably will not see much improvement in the quality of the handwriting.

Most children and teens with poor handwriting can improve to the point where homework is no longer a problem. As with everything we want our children to learn, the first stage is teaching them <u>how</u> to do it correctly. Then we need to train them so that they develop the <u>habit</u> of doing it correctly.

Preparing the environment for improved handwriting

- For all handwriting practice, have your child use a pencil, rather than a pen, so that he can rub out. The more you Descriptively Praise the letters that are just right or almost right, the sooner he will notice for himself the letters which are not quite right. He will want to rub them out and write them correctly. For very young children, chalk or large crayons are easier to manage than pencils.

- Many schools use unlined paper in Reception, possibly because they think young children do not yet have the fine-motor control needed to keep their letters on the line. In my experience, this is not true. The right kind of handwriting paper can be very helpful for teaching children where to position their letters and guiding them into good habits. However, ordinary lined paper does not provide children with the guidance they need when they are practising handwriting.

A young child who is just learning to write tends to make letters very large. Giving her squared paper with quite large boxes teaches her that letters have to be a certain size to fit in the box. As she masters writing letters in the large boxes, you can make the boxes progressively smaller.

Putting letters on the line is often easier for children to understand and master than getting the shape or size right. So Descriptively Praise whenever your child happens to write a letter on the line.

- Once your child has mastered keeping her letters inside a relatively small box and on the line, the next step is to use lined paper with a halfway line that is a different colour. That helps children focus on keeping the small letters small, going up only to the halfway line.

- We need to make sure that the child's feet are resting flat on the floor. This gives his whole body the stability to maintain a straight back. When children's feet dangle, their posture is often slumped over, and their handwriting suffers.

Some of the activities that I suggest in this section may strike you as too babyish for an older child or teen, possibly even insulting. Please don't be put off by how basic these exercises may seem. Judge for yourself whether your child needs practice with a particular skill, rather than being swayed by your child's complaints. These activities work to improve handwriting, so if handwriting is a problem, be willing to do them. Everyone will feel better when your child's handwriting improves.

The ten-minute handwriting lesson

Start each day's homework session with a short handwriting lesson — no more than ten minutes. This will result in the homework that follows being done more carefully (although not perfectly, of course). Your child or teen may protest, but persevere. Descriptive Praise, Reflective Listening and Preparing for Success will all help to reduce resistance.

Whenever we are guiding children to improve a skill, we need to start at their current skill level and work up as they demonstrate mastery, rather than starting where we wish they were or where the rest of the class is. You can easily assess whether your child can write all her letters correctly by having her write the alphabet, both lower-case and upper-case.

Improving spatial awareness

The very first step in improving your child's handwriting does not actually involve your child doing any writing! It's all about improving spatial awareness. You may have read about how ordinary people, who do not consider themselves to be at all artistic, have learnt to draw faces to a very high standard by being taught about the actual proportions of a face. We tend, for example, to assume that eyes should be drawn towards the top of the head, whereas in fact they are in the middle of the head. Similarly, pointing out to children the correct shapes and sizes of letters rapidly improves their handwriting.

To improve spatial awareness, make letter tiles out of card, and show your child the characteristics of different letters by grouping together all the letters that are tall or all the letters that hang down or all that have a circle or a stick or that look almost the same (such as *n* and *h*, which differ only in the height of the stick or *r* and *n*, which differ only in where the arch ends). You can improve your child's spatial awareness by using the letter tiles to show which upper-case and lower-case letters look the same except for size (eg *c, o, p, s, v, w, x* and *z*) and which upper-case and lower-case letters are almost the same (eg *f, I, j, k, t, u, y*). You can show which pairs of letters can be mistaken for each other if not written correctly (eg *e* and *i* or *a* and *u* or *g* and *y*).

Show your child that we start writing each letter from the top of the letter. For small letters that means starting at the halfway line.

You can also buy what are called sandpaper letters. These use the child's tactile sense to teach him the shape of the letters and the direction in which they are written.

Lastly, make a game of finding, in magazines and news-papers, examples of the letters you have been teaching him about.

Practising writing under your supervision

Once your child knows and can point out and describe the characteristics of all the letters, the next stage is for him to practise writing while you supervise closely. We are aiming for error-free learning so that the correct way to write each letter is what is stored in the child's long-term memory. We do not want children to practise their mistakes because that would be counter-productive.

To maximise the likelihood of error-free learning, first we need to do *think-throughs*. The kinds of questions you might ask during a one minute *think-through* are:

*How will you make sure that your **e** looks like an **e** and your **i** looks like an **i**?*

Which letters in the alphabet hang down?

Which letters in your name are tall letters?

Then we need to pay attention while the child writes so that we can Descriptively Praise everything he is doing right, even if the improvement is not as much as we would like to see:

All the letters in this word are sitting on the line.

*I can tell this letter is a **g** and not a **y** because you closed the circle.*

*You made a tall **t**.*

We also need to intervene immediately when we see him writing incorrectly, for example, writing a capital letter the same size as lower-case letters or drifting below the line. Use a *diagnostic response* (see Chapter 11) to show your child what his mistake is:

*You remembered to make a dot for your **i**, but you made it so close to the stick that I can hardly see it.*

During the ten-minute handwriting lesson, children should be writing words or sentences that interest them. Young children are usually keen to write their own name and also the names of other family members, and this is a good opportunity to make sure they can spell their full names. Names of animals are often popular. Have a young child trace over letters that you have written. You could also combine handwriting practice with spelling practice by having children write their weekly spelling words. When the size of your child's writing is a problem, put a small coloured dot on the page to show where he should start the letter.

Correcting an ineffective pencil grip

Children frequently develop an incorrect pencil grip, which can hamper their handwriting and even in some cases cause physical discomfort. Teachers often advise parents not to try and change an incorrect pencil grip on the grounds that it will not work and will just frustrate the child. This is not accurate. An incorrect grip can be corrected at any age, once your child or teen is motivated. Have your child practise the correct pencil grip during the short handwriting lesson that comes before each day's homework. You will need to insist on this and be vigilant. Make sure to Descriptively Praise the correct pencil grip and Reflectively Listen if your child complains at first that the new way of holding the pencil feels uncomfortable. Have your child practise the new pencil grip as he pretends to write in the air. This will get his hand accustomed to how the new position of his fingers feels without the discomfort that he may feel when he first starts to write.

Improving eye-hand coordination

To help a child improve eye-hand coordination, start with large movements that use the whole arm. This will be easier than small movements, which use only the muscles in the hand. To use the whole arm, have your child pretend to write letters in the air, holding the pencil correctly. He can graduate to writing large letters on a very large piece of paper, such as an old newspaper. Write letters in black marker and have your child trace them, first with his index finger, then with a thick crayon or marker and finally with a pencil.

Keep the cars on the road

This game is useful for teaching eye-hand coordination. The parent draws two straight parallel lines. The child's job is to move the 'car', which is the pencil, along the road, staying within the parallel lines. With practice your child's eye-hand coordination will improve, and you will be able to make 'the road' narrower and put in twists and turns.

Dot-to-dot

The parent draws the shape of a letter in dots, and the child has to write the letter by joining up the dots. For this exercise to be useful, the child has to put his pencil through every dot without taking any short cuts. Writing letters that have sharp corners is difficult for young children or for those with weak fine motor skills, so make sure that the dots at the angles of letters do not get missed out.

Independent writing

The third stage in improving handwriting is for your child to practise independently, with you just giving feedback at the end. Only move on to this stage when your child is writing mostly correctly while you are monitoring.

Teaching and improving joined-up writing

Some schools start by teaching children how to print. Others teach children how to put a 'flick' (the technical term for this is an exit stroke) at the end of each letter in preparation for the time when they will be joining up the letters. This is a sensible strategy because children are learning from the beginning what they will need eventually, rather than learning one set of letters and later having to learn a whole new set. Once the exit strokes have been mastered, then schools usually introduce the entrance strokes. For these, the pencil starts on the line and then goes up to make the letter. This can be confusing for children because the entrance stroke is intended only for joining letters within a word, not for the first letter of a word. I recommend not teaching the entrance stroke. When your child starts to learn joined-up writing, simply show him how the flick of one letter is used to attach that letter to the next.

Many children who have mastered printing find the transition to joined-up writing quite difficult. This is often because they have to control their pencil for a whole word, whereas with printing they are focusing on only one letter at a time. To bridge the gap between writing individual letters in print and writing whole words in joined-up, start by having children practise joining up only two letters at a time. You could start for example with *at, ap, as, an, al*, etc. Your child is learning how to join the *a* to every other letter. Make sure that this knowledge is solid before you go on to teach your child how to join up another letter.

Once children are skilled in joined up writing, their writing looks more grown-up, so they feel proud. And with practice they will be able to write more quickly, which becomes important when they have to take notes.

Improving handwriting during homework

Everything I have talked about so far is for the short handwriting lesson that comes before the daily homework session. Now I want to talk about how to handle handwriting during homework.

Stage One is the *think-through*. You will be asking questions to bring back into the child's short-term memory what she needs to be focusing on in order to do her best rather than to simply practise her earlier mistakes. In addition to asking questions about what she will write and about spelling, punctuation, etc., also ask questions about pencil grip, about the size of letters, the shape of letters, where the letters are supposed to sit, etc.

In Stage Two your child does the homework independently, with no correcting from you. Please do notice and Descriptively Praise any small improvements in handwriting, as well as in spelling, punctuation, vocabulary, etc. For a very young child, Stage One can include his dictating a sentence to you that he then copies in his own writing in Stage Two.

In Stage Three, which is the improving stage, both you and your child will first look for and find bits of the writing to Descriptively Praise. This is an important exercise. Children learn a great deal from paying attention to what they have done right. When it is time to notice and mention the two things that your child needs to correct, I recommend <u>not</u> focusing on handwriting mistakes. The short handwriting lesson that precedes the homework is a much more effective way of improving handwriting. In Stage Three, choose other types of mistakes to mention, such as an inaccuracy or a spelling mistake or an answer that is incomplete.

In addition to the short handwriting lesson that precedes the daily homework time and the writing that happens during homework, your child may write spontaneously at other times. He may write a list or a card to a friend; he may choose on his own to write a story or a poem. Do not correct his handwriting in these situations because you do not want to put him off this spontaneous writing. Instead, simply Descriptively Praise as much as possible.

CHAPTER 20

IMPROVING EDITING AND PROOFREADING SKILLS

Both of my children were fairly good students. But the big problem was that they couldn't be bothered to check their work. So the quality of it ended up being much poorer than it should have been. After years of me ranting and raving about it, the solution was to break each piece of homework into the three stages, the way Noël says. Why didn't I do this sooner! In Stage One I asked lots of think-through questions about proofreading. And in Stage Three I started pointing out the good things in their work. I'm embarrassed to admit that I hadn't ever really done that before. My wife and I used to focus on the things they did wrong and lecture them. Before I started our new plan, I thought they wouldn't want to correct anything in Stage Three. But there are always only four mistakes to correct, so they're willing. The other thing we did was in the holidays I used to play a game with them that Noël recommends, where each person writes a sentence with a certain number of mistakes and the other person has to find and correct the mistakes. They loved that game because they could put in some hilarious mistakes! It was fun and they learned a lot about proofreading from that game. It sometimes seems like a miracle, but now our boys are both very good students, and they like school so much more. They want to do good work, and they're proud of their stories and essays. I'm so grateful I came across all these strategies.

Father of two teenagers, aged 15 and 13

As adults, we know that our first attempt at anything is rarely our very best effort. When we need to write anything important (our CV, a report for work, a letter of complaint), we always proofread and improve our first draft, often rewriting it several times. Children need to learn this process and develop the habit of proofreading. Some will fall into this habit quite easily, whilst others, usually the more impulsive, impatient ones, will resist, either actively or passively. Some children manage to defeat the best efforts of parents and teachers to motivate and encourage them to pay attention to the details that need improving. It seems as if they just can't be bothered to slow down. But that is not really the whole story.

It takes these children a long time to learn how to proofread effectively, and even after they know how, they may do it sketchily. Of course, this affects their marks at school and even, over time, their self-esteem because they are reprimanded so frequently. They come to see themselves as lazy or stupid. However, these children can be trained to edit, expand and proofread carefully in order to improve their written work.

The responsibility for this training will usually fall on parents because teachers rarely have the time. Parents need to view this training as an ongoing project. It will take time and determination. There are two ways to teach and train these skills, and both are needed:

- During homework
- Outside of homework, during activities designed to target specific micro-skills

Does your child know how to improve her work?

When we explain anything to children before finding out what they already know and can do, we risk underestimating and possibly insulting them (and wasting our time and theirs). Or we may unwittingly pitch our explanations over their head, which leads to even more confusion, resentment and discouragement. Before you start training and teaching, make sure you have spent time exploring what your child already knows or thinks he knows (which are often not the same thing at all).

Do not assume that your child knows how to proofread accurately but is simply being careless or 'lazy'. What is much more likely is that he has not yet mastered the micro-skills necessary for improving his written work:

- Teach (and revise frequently) the use of a spelling dictionary and a computer spellchecker.
- Choose a user-friendly dictionary for checking meanings.
- Teach the use of a thesaurus for enriching vocabulary.
- Have your child, under your guidance, refer to a simple grammar book for rules governing punctuation.
- In daily conversation, frequently point out formal versus informal sentence construction so that your child comes to understand that what is acceptable in speech is often not acceptable in writing.
- When you are talking with your child, model and guide him to practise clear sentence construction.
- Descriptively Praise attention to detail in everything, not just homework.

Improving the quality of written work takes time

We need to distinguish between two different goals. One is teaching and training the techniques necessary for improving proofreading and editing skills. This is the parents' job. The other is getting the child's homework corrected before he hands it in to the teacher. That should <u>not</u> be our goal. If it is our goal, we may be tempted to save time and hassle by telling him how to improve his work. Instead, we need to take the time to guide him to discover for himself what needs to be corrected and why and how.

Sometimes parents end up doing their child's thinking for them because they feel 'the work must get done'. This is a fallacy! Learning takes as long as it takes. So we <u>cannot</u> and <u>must not</u> assume that a child will finish a certain amount of work by seven pm or that he will reach a certain standard by the end of the term. Our job as parents is to teach and train the important skills, concepts, attitudes, habits and values. We can never accurately predict how long it will take a child to master these.

First steps for improving proofreading and editing skills

Regularly discuss with your child how even the greatest authors do not expect to be able to produce work they are pleased with the first time.

In fact, the process of editing and proofreading is what results in good writing. So there is absolutely no shame attached to having to improve one's first draft.

Whenever you can, model the desired proofreading behaviour.

Let your child see you proofreading your own writing, even if it's just a shopping list or a sentence or two on a quick note. Muse aloud to show what the thought processes involved are:

Hmmm, I wonder if I spelled that right. I'll look it up to make sure.

Should this be colon or a semicolon? Actually, maybe it would sound better if I made these into two separate sentences. Now how does that sound? Yes, much better.

Talk often with your children about how writing, editing and proofreading are all different skills and they each use a different part of the brain. Children are often fascinated to learn how their minds work.

Using homework to teach and train proofreading and editing skills

1 **The daily homework *think-through* in Stage One (see Chapter 5) is the first step in teaching and training proofreading and editing.**
   Think-throughs teach and train the child to monitor his work as he is producing it. And because *think-throughs* always result in a higher standard of homework, the child is then much more willing, during Stage Three, to tackle the smaller number of errors.

2 **Whenever there is enough time, require each piece of writing homework to be done in rough first.** Knowing that the first draft will be rough enables your child to relax and focus on getting his ideas down, without his brain being burdened by the need to keep in his working memory the details of punctuation, capital letters, spelling and handwriting. You may be concerned that writing both a rough and a final copy would take too much time. Interestingly, it usually saves time. Children and teens soon come to enjoy writing a rough draft, once they realise that they are temporarily freed from the drudgery or anxiety of attention to

detail. Even die-hard avoiders of writing waste less time getting started and often whiz through the rough draft.

- Have your child skip alternate lines on the page for all rough work. This double-spacing leaves room for corrections and additions.

- Have your child use a pencil for all rough work. Encourage crossing out rather than rubbing out so that the flow of his thoughts is not interrupted.

- While your child is writing, either the rough draft or the final copy, do not correct, advise, prompt, nudge, point, raise your eyebrows or say, 'Are you sure?'

- The exception to this policy of a rough draft would be exam practice, where the writing needs to be done under exam-type conditions.

- Eventually (but this will take longer to achieve than you would like), a rough draft will not always be necessary because your child will learn to edit and proofread his writing <u>as he writes</u> resulting, over time, in a better and better standard of work.

3 **You may find that your child's writing style is vague or garbled, padded or repetitive, too flowery or simply very patchy and immature.**

Do not let him attempt piecemeal corrections directly onto his rough draft. His paper will end up a confusing and discouraging mess. If you know that your child's writing is likely to have these faults, don't let him get started in the same old way. Instead, he will need to be taught how to simplify and clarify his points. This is best done starting from scratch. The following three steps will teach your child to write more clearly:

1. Have your child tell you what he wants to write while you jot down each point briefly, clearly and neatly in

note form on only one side of individual pieces of paper. Children can speak better than they can write, and they are more confident when they are speaking, so this step alone eliminates a lot of the problem.

2. Then have your child rearrange the pieces of paper until he is happy with the order in which he wants to make his points.

3. Finally, your child's job is to write one or more sentences for each of his points.

Over time, these three steps will result in a cleaner, more mature style of written expression. This technique also works whenever a child is stuck. Even a child who can think of nothing to write can usually talk about the topic if the parent asks 'wh' questions: *who, what, when, where, why, how* and *which*.

4 **If possible, separate in time the writing stage from the improving stage.**

Whenever you can, wait until the next day before coming back to the work for the improving stage. If that is not possible, a short break is better than none. It allows the child's brain to shift function from creating to evaluating.

5 **Once the rough draft is completed, put lots of your time and attention during Stage 3 into finding and appreciating all the good things about it.**

Children and teenagers (and adults!) are usually very attentive when they are hearing good things about themselves. Your child will learn far more from hearing about what she has done right than from hearing about what she should have done differently. When children feel criticised, they tend (as any of us would) to get annoyed and defensive or to feel ashamed or to switch off altogether. None of those reactions result in much learning.

You can Descriptively Praise any examples you see of accuracy, thoroughness, interesting style or vocabulary that is more mature or particularly vivid. And you will want to use the power of your Descriptive Praise to reinforce any improvements in spelling, punctuation or use of capital letters. Be very specific in your Descriptive Praise:

> You've used some very technical words in this essay and you explained each one. Even someone who has no knowledge of the topic, like me, can understand.

> You've put a capital letter for every single proper noun. Now I can easily tell who's who.

> From the words you used to describe the soldier, I can really imagine how he must have felt.

> You've really mastered full stops. There isn't a single run-on sentence in this whole essay!

You may remember that in Chapter 5 I explained that in Stage 3, the improving stage, your child will have a maximum of four corrections to make on each piece of homework. However, when you are teaching and training proofreading skills, your child will be practising finding as many things as possible to correct or improve.

6 **With your child, generate a checklist of all the aspects of the work that need checking.**
Do this each time your child is about to proofread and edit a new piece of work, rather than referring to a

previous checklist. By *attempting to retrieve* the elements that need to be checked, your child will start to memorise and internalise these points.

Then discuss with your child which of these aspects of writing he will proofread and in which order. Let the ideas come from him. Be willing to wait for his contributions. Find something to Descriptively Praise or agree with in each idea your child offers. Avoid saying, 'But . . .' Keep a list of the useful points that come out of this discussion.

7 **Make your child's brain do the work.**
Do not fall into the trap of answering questions that your child could figure out for himself or look up. He may need support with this process, and it will certainly be slower than if you simply told him or explained it. But he will learn and remember much more if it is <u>his</u> brain that does the work.

Have him tell you what the corrections should be and why. If we tell him what's wrong and then he corrects his mistakes, we may convince him, and possibly even ourselves, that his relatively error-free final draft is actually his work. It is not. It is, at best, a sort of collaboration. This is not what schools have in mind when they set homework! Homework is designed to be the child's work.

At first, to make it easier for your child to find his mistakes, you can use a system that lets him know how many mistakes there are of each type on each line. For example, you can jot 'sp' in the margin if there is a word misspelled on that line. Then he needs to use his own brain to pinpoint that mistake.

To make the corrections easier for your child to decipher when it is time to write out his final copy, both you and your child should use a coloured pen for marking the changes. Avoid red, which often has negative associations.

8 **Descriptively Praise your child for finding errors.**
Be glad, and show that you're glad, that he found the errors, rather than being annoyed that he made the errors in the first place. Make it clear that the whole point of proofreading is to discover errors, not to find that there are no errors.

9 **Even when you're drawing your child's attention to an error, practise making your point through Descriptive Praise.**
You could say:

> *You've written seven sentences here, and five of them start with a capital letter. You've put capitals at the beginning of almost all of your sentences.*

> *Your handwriting is so much easier to read now that you're keeping most of the letters on the line.*

> *You've got all the right letters here. You just need to put them in the right order.*

10 **When there is time, have your child proofread his rough draft several times.**
Each time have him look for a different type of error:
- Content
  1. Choice of topic
  2. Organisation of ideas
  3. Development of ideas
  4. Length
  5. Sentence construction

- Vocabulary
- Spelling
- Punctuation
- Capital letters

Have your child read through his work, at a leisurely pace, looking for mistakes in each one of these aspects at a time, with your child doing the thinking, the explaining and the correcting. Concentrate on the aspects that most need improvement.

11 **The final draft of homework should be executed in exactly the way the school requires.**
Most teachers have their own rules about how to write the heading, what and how to underline, whether tippex is permitted, crossings out, insertions, etc. If a disagreement or question about acceptable presentation arises during Stages One or Three of the homework session, use <u>your</u> best judgement rather than simply taking your child's word for it. Then make a note to yourself to find out from the school exactly how they want it to be done.

12 **Always end the proofreading or editing part of the homework session on an up note, with lots of Descriptive Praise.**

13 **Always take a minute at the end of each homework session to jot down which proofreading points have just been revised and which need to be revised.**
It is easy to make the mistake of concentrating on certain aspects and ignoring other aspects.

14 **When you are using your child's homework as the vehicle for teaching proofreading, remember to indicate, for the school's information, how much and**

what type of help or instruction you gave your child.
Otherwise the teachers may be mystified or suspicious if
his writing has suddenly improved. The best way to keep
teachers informed is to send the rough draft back to school
along with the final copy.

Proofreading for spelling

Teaching children and teens how to proofread for spelling does
more than improve the quality of their work, important though
that is. Proofreading also teaches children a lot about <u>how</u> to
spell and trains them in the <u>habit</u> of thinking about spelling.
There are a number of useful ways to tackle proofreading for
spelling. I recommend you experiment with all of them.

- To help your child learn how to proofread a piece of homework for spelling, make a list of all the words containing
  five or more letters that are spelled <u>correctly</u> in the rough
  draft of his essay. He then checks his work to see which
  words from his writing have been left off your list. To
  compare the words in his rough draft with those on your
  list, he has to pay attention to several pieces of information at the same time, which will, over time, improve his
  working memory. As he identifies and corrects the
  misspelled words, you then add them to the list of
  correctly spelled words. Seeing this list grow as he corrects
  his mistakes is highly motivating for most children, especially if you team it with lots of Descriptive Praise.
- In addition, keep an ongoing list (which will change over
  time) of words that your child frequently misspells. Have
  him circle these words in his rough draft and then
  compare his spellings to the list.

- When there is time, have your child check the spelling of every word in his work that has more than five letters, or six or seven. First have him go through his story or essay and circle all those words, then go back and look them up.
- When checking for spelling, have your child read the words out of context, for example by reading the piece of writing backwards, word by word. This will counter the natural tendency to 'see' what one wants or expects to see, rather than what is really written on the page.
- Take the time to help your child notice why he misspelled a word. With practice, this *diagnostic response* (see Chapter 11) will give him the necessary tools to think about spelling as he proofreads (and eventually as he writes). Most spelling mistakes are caused by only nine types of errors:

  - Missing out a silent letter (*anser* for *answer*, *bred* for *bread*)
  - Not understanding the rule for when to double the consonant before adding *ing* or *ed* and when not to (*slidding* for *sliding* or *triped* for *tripped*)
  - Confusion between words that look or sound similar (*went* looks very much like *want*; *except* sounds like *accept*)
  - Not remembering which vowel combinations makes the long-vowel sound in which words (eg *treet* for *treat* or *tale* for *tail*)
  - Writing all the right letters but in the wrong order (*gril* for *girl* or *brian* for *brain*)
  - Leaving off *ed* when writing in the past tense (*he walk* for *he walked*)
  - Confusing the spelling of words that sound identical, but have different meanings (*to, too, two* or *there, their, they're*)
  - Attempting to spell words or syllables phonetically

that are not spelled phonetically (*moove* for *move* or *shun* for *tion*)

- Omitting the *silent e* that 'makes the vowel say its name' (writing *hop* for *hope*) or over-generalising and adding a *silent e* where it serves no purpose (*hande* for *hand*)

In Chapter 18, I explain some very effective strategies for helping children to become better spellers.

Proofreading for punctuation and capital letters

When proofreading for punctuation and capital letters, have your child proofread in stages. First, check carefully for capital letters at the beginnings of sentences and for proper nouns. Next, for full stops, question marks or exclamation points at the ends of sentences. Then have him proofread for apostrophes, then for commas and finally for quotation marks.

Beware! Commas are very problematic, and acceptable usage can differ from school to school, even from teacher to teacher. So before asking your child to add or remove a comma, make sure that you know what rules he must abide by.

To summarise, proofreading can feel terrible for children (and for parents) if we get annoyed about 'careless' mistakes. We need to remember that carelessness is often a learned response, the result of habitual avoidance or rushing. When we take the time to teach and train proofreading as I have outlined in this chapter, the child's willingness to pay attention to details improves, as well as his ability to do so. Proofreading may never become his favourite activity, but it can become much, much easier. You will see his confidence blossom as he starts to take pride in his work.

CONCLUSION

Last year I had a very tricky class. They were much more difficult than usual — problems with not concentrating, problems with not following directions, problems with doing their homework very poorly or not even bothering to do it at all. And they didn't get better as the year progressed; they actually seemed to be getting worse. I was at my wits' end. I'd been to some seminars at the Calmer, Easier, Happier Parenting Centre, so I already knew about the five core strategies. And I knew they worked with my grandchildren, but I hadn't really thought about using them in my classroom. But I decided it was worth a try so I put into practice the homework techniques Noël recommends. I actually taught them how to do their homework properly. And I taught the Calmer, Easier, Happier Homework rules and routines to any parent who would listen. And this may seem like it couldn't be true, but my class went from having the worst reputation in the school to being considered the easiest class. It took about a term, and it wasn't always easy, but it felt so good. Their behaviour improved and also the quality of their work, what they did in class and their homework. I now know that these strategies that Noël talks about can help all children improve their behaviour and their learning and their motivation, even the children with learning difficulties and even the defiant and distractible ones that were driving me up the wall.

A teacher, Year Seven

Once you start putting the Calmer, Easier, Happier Homework rules and routines into practice, you will very quickly notice small, subtle improvements in attitude, attention span, attention to detail and learning — often within days, certainly within weeks. As with practising any new routine or learning any new skill, the first few weeks are likely to be the hardest, for you as well as for your children. But if you stick with this plan, within a few short months you will see significant progress. For most children, the Calmer, Easier, Happier Homework plan will be all that is needed to get their learning and their self-confidence back on track.

But for some children, usually those with more severe problems, more help may be necessary. When looking for help from professionals, parents are easily confused because there are many different ways that a child with school or homework problems can be assessed and helped. Some of these interventions are well known and widely respected. Others are as yet less well understood and less popular. In order to help a child fulfil his potential, parents can pursue remedial tutoring, conventional therapies, alternative treatments and medical interventions. For almost every approach you choose to explore, you will discover some parents who have found it very helpful for their child and some parents who did not see much improvement.

From my own investigations, I have experienced that all interventions work best when parents commit to establishing enjoyable and productive homework habits. So whichever additional approach you may choose to explore, give it a fighting chance to make a real difference in your child's life. Persevere with the Calmer, Easier, Happier Homework rules and routines. If you are wondering whether there might be any incompatibility between these strategies and any other approach you are interested in exploring, simply show this book to the professionals in question, and they will advise you.

I am hoping that by now you are feeling empowered to get back in charge of your children's learning and behaviour. Remember:

> Our children's education is far too important to leave up to the schools.

So get started and keep going. It won't always be plain sailing. But week by week and month by month you will see that the more positive, firm and consistent you remain, the calmer, easier and happier homework will become. As you put these strategies into practice, you will be guiding your children to fulfil their potential – an invaluable gift that all parents want to be able to give their children.

THE MOST USEFUL WORD LIST OF ALL

Following is a list of the 221 most common words in English-language books. These words make up seventy percent of all the words your child will be reading and writing. If parents and teachers were to focus on teaching children to read and spell these words accurately and quickly, think how much calmer, easier and happier homework would be!

Group One: These twelve words make up approximately twenty-five percent of all reading

a	it
and	of
he	that
I	the
in	to
is	was

Group Two: These twenty words, added to the first group, make up approximately thirty-three percent of all reading

all	be	have	on	they
are	but	him	one	we
as	for	his	said	with
at	had	not	so	you

Group Three: This group of 70 words completes the 102 words that make up an average of fifty percent of all reading

about	look	two
an	made	up
back	make	want
been	more	well
before	me	went
big	much	were
by	must	what
call	my	when
came	no	where
can	new	which
come	now	who
could	off	will
did	old	yes
do	only	your
down	or	
first	other	
from	our	
gave	out	
get	over	
go	right	
has	see	
her	she	
here	some	
if	their	
into	them	
just	then	
like	there	
little	this	

Group Four: These 119 words, added to the above words, make up seventy percent of all reading and writing

after	fall	let	sleep	would
again	for	light	small	write
always	fast	live	soon	yellow
any	find	long	start	
around	five	may	stop	
ask	fly	myself	take	
ate	found	never	tell	
away	four	once	ten	
because	full	open	thank	
best	funny	own	these	
better	gave	pick	think	
black	give	play	those	
blue	goes	please	three	
both	going	pretty	today	
bring	good	pull	together	
brown	got	put	too	
buy	green	ran	try	
carry	grow	read	under	
clean	help	red	upon	
cold	hold	ride	us	
cut	hot	round	use	
does	how	run	very	
done	hurt	saw	walk	
don't	its	seven	warm	
draw	jump	shall	wash	
drink	keep	show	while	
eat	kind	sing	why	
eight	know	sit	wish	
every	laugh	six	work	

RESOURCES

Noël Janis-Norton is the director of the Calmer, Easier, Happier Parenting Centre, a not-for-profit consultancy that works worldwide with families and with professionals who work with families.

The staff of certified parenting practitioners includes parent coaches, family coaches and group facilitators.

The Centre offers the following services:
Introductory talks for parents (at the Centre, in schools and in the workplace)
Parenting skills courses
Seminars and webinars
Private sessions (at the Centre, by telephone or in the home)
School visits to observe a child and guide teachers
Mediation between parents
Teacher-training

In addition, the Centre offers a wide range of products: books, audio-CDs and DVDs on many aspects of parenting and teaching.

CDs about the five core strategies of Calmer, Easier, Happier Parenting:

1   Descriptive Praise
2   Preparing for Success
3   Reflective Listening
4   Never Ask Twice
5   Rewards and Consequences

Topic CD sets:

Siblings with Less Rivalry (3 discs)
Calmer, Easier, Happier Mealtimes (2 discs)
Calmer, Easier, Happier Music Practice (2 discs)
Bringing Out the Best in Children and Teens with Special Needs
    (5 discs)

DVDs:

Bringing Out the Best in Boys
Transforming Homework Hassles

Books for parents:

Calmer, Easier, Happier Parenting by Noël Janis-Norton
Could Do Better by Noël Janis-Norton
How to Calm a Challenging Child by Miriam Chachamu
How to Be a Better Parent by Cassandra Jardine
Positive Not Pushy by Cassandra Jardine
Where Has My Little Girl Gone? by Tanith Carey

Books for teachers:

In Step with Your Class by Noël Janis-Norton
Learning to Listen, Listening to Learn by Noël Janis-Norton

For more information about the Calmer, Easier, Happier Parenting resources, please visit the following websites:

www.calmerparenting.co.uk (**UK**)

www.calmerparenting.com (**North America**)

www.calmerparenting.fr (**France**)

INDEX